Being Black in My Family

By ChaQuana McEntyre

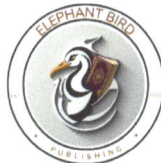

Elephant Bird Publishing

Duluth, MN | Dallas, TX

Being Black in My Family

By ChaQuana McEntyre

Published by Elephant Bird Publishing

ISBN: 979-8-9928901-2-9

Printed in the United States of America

To order copies of this book or to book a training for your organization, please contact Family Rise Together via phone at +1-218-390-9204 or the website **FamilyRiseTogether.org** for more info.

10 9 8 7 6 CQME 5 4 3 2 1

Dedication Page

This book is for the black children who are cherished yet often feel invisible in the place they call home. For the ones who, in the depths of their souls, wrestle with a quiet, unshakable sense of not belonging.

To the seven-year-old ChaQuana McEntyre Jones, LuCretia Jones, and Sade Sandidge—this is for you.

I see you.
We see each other.

CM Jones

A Note From
the Author

Dear Reader,

Thank you for spending time with Being Black in My Family. I wrote this book for kids just like you—kids who might have big questions, mixed feelings, and beautiful, unique families. I want you to know something very important: you are not alone.

Your identity is not confusing—it's complex, powerful, and worth celebrating. Being Black is not about how others define you—it's about how you feel, what you choose to embrace, and the stories you carry in your heart.

It's okay to have questions. It's okay to feel proud and unsure sometimes. That's part of growing. Just remember: you are whole. You are worthy. And you belong.

To the caregivers and adults reading this: thank you for showing up for the children in your life. Keep listening. Keep learning. And know that your presence matters more than perfection ever could.

With love and hope,

C.M. Jones

Author of Being Black in My Family

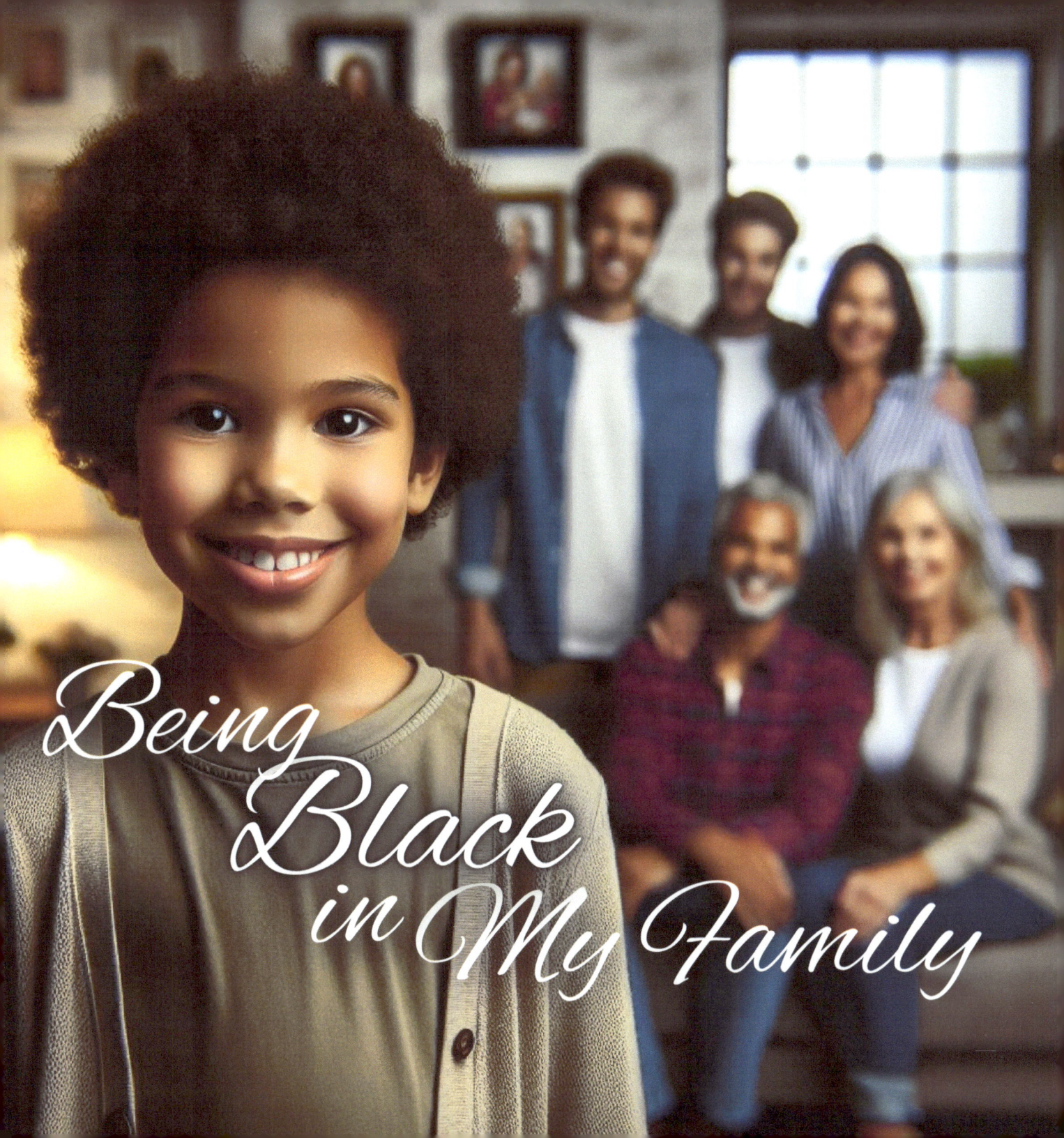

Being
Black
in My Family

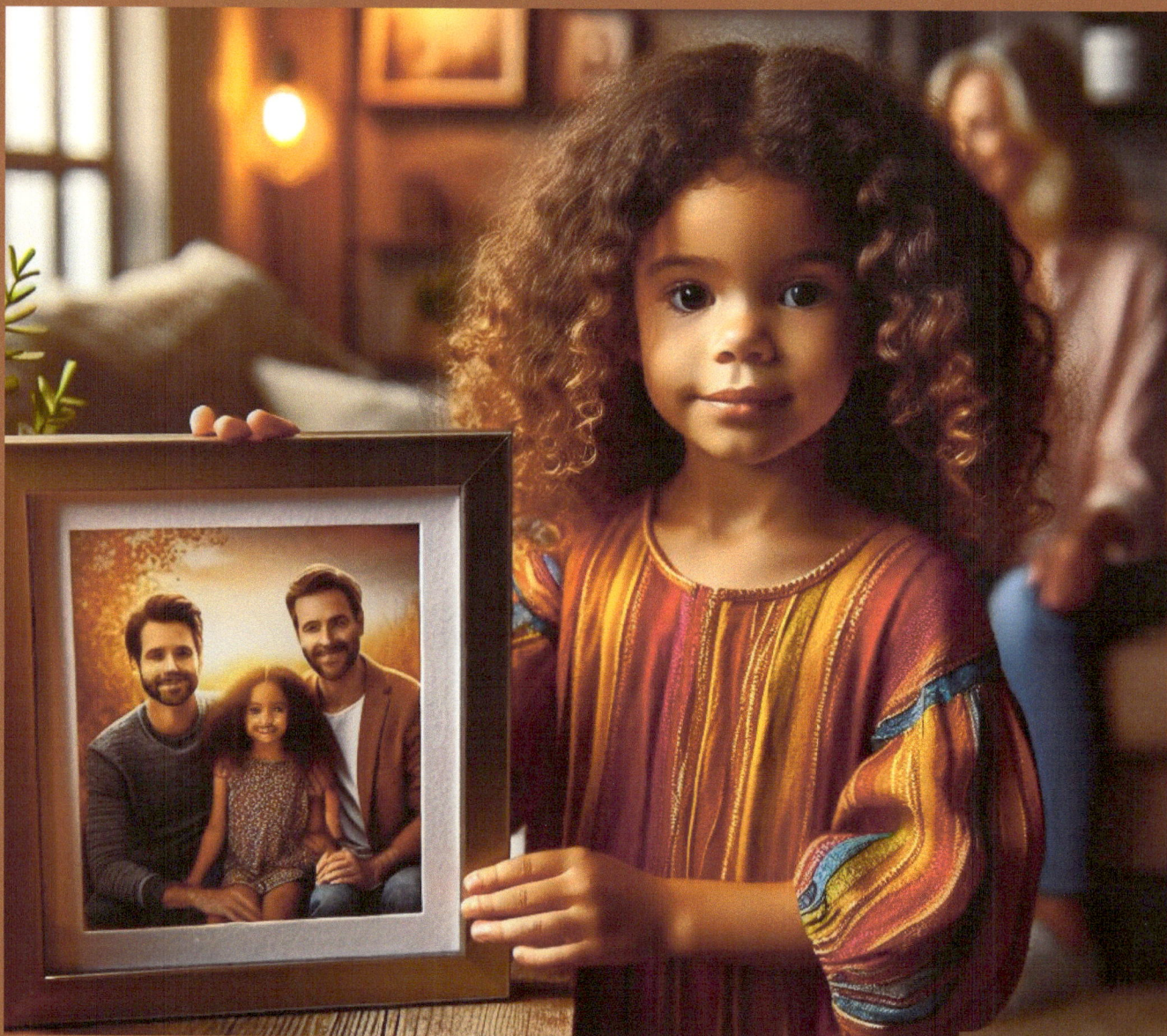

My name is _____, and I am Black.

But in my family,

I am the only one who looks like me.

Sometimes, that makes me feel special.

Other times, it makes me feel different.

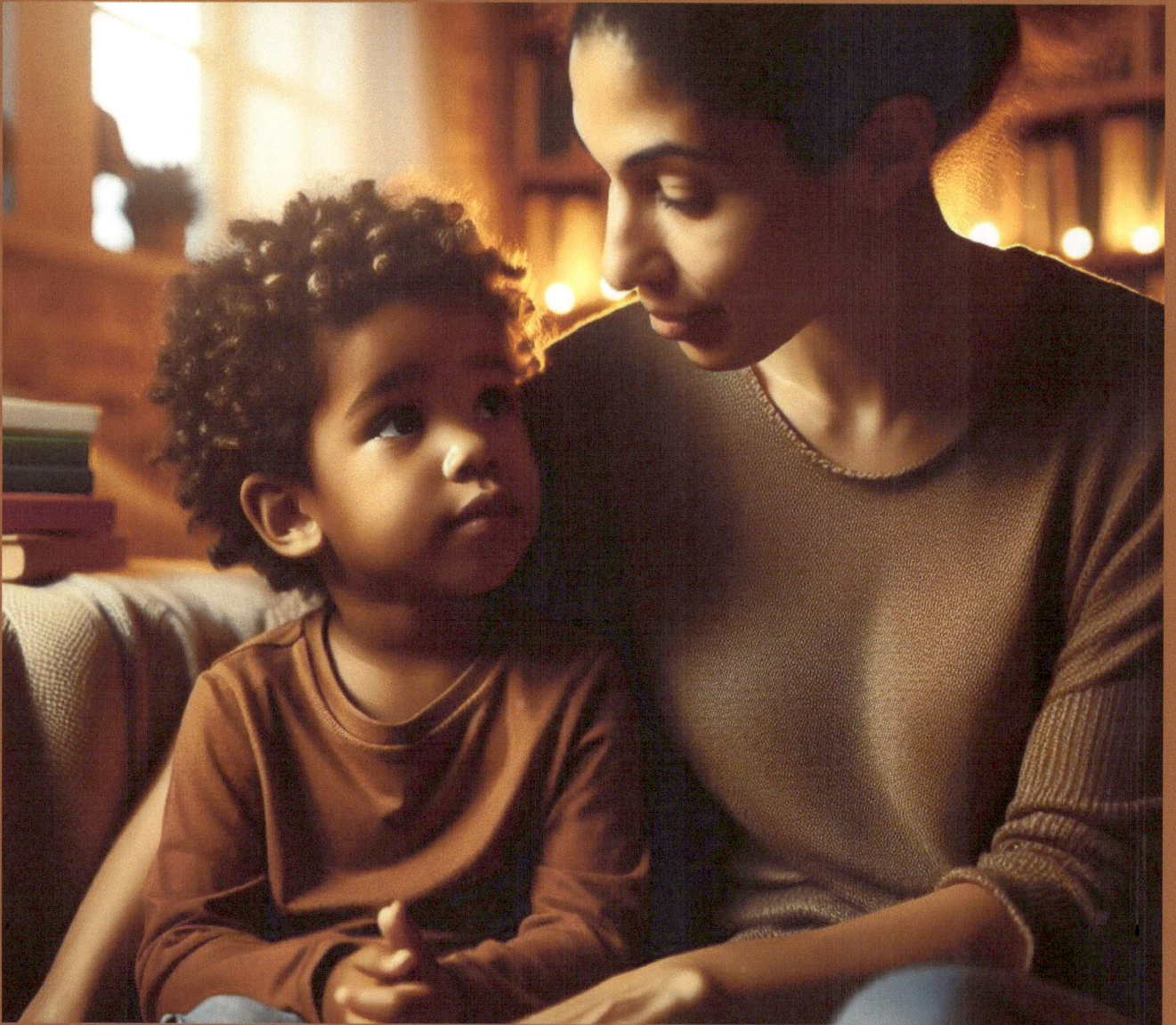

My mom loves me so much.

But sometimes, I wonder if they really understand what it's like to be me.

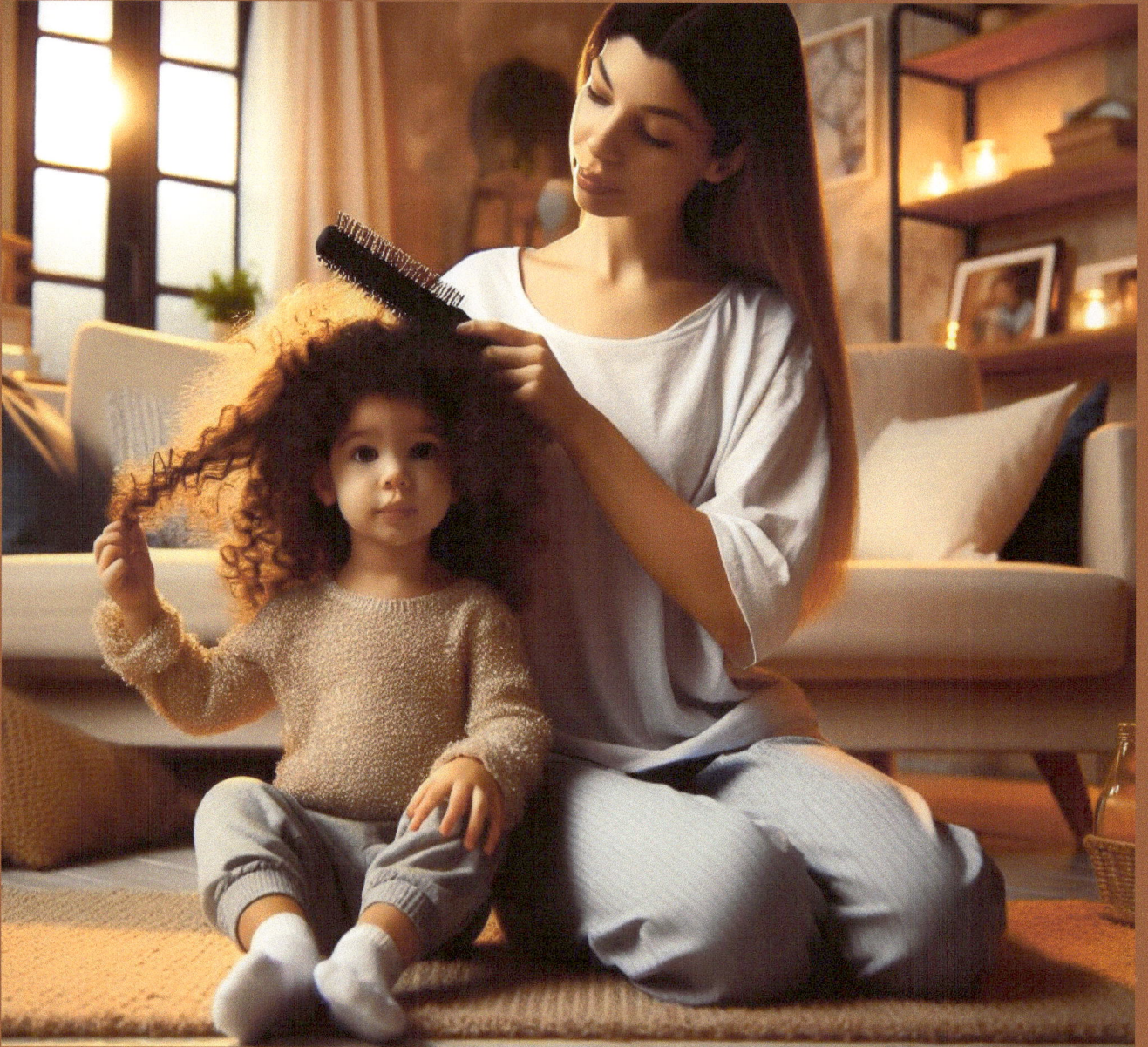

One of the things I wonder about is my hair.

My curls twist and turn in ways my mom's (or dad's) hair never does. It feels soft like cotton, but sometimes it tangles and takes a long time to comb.

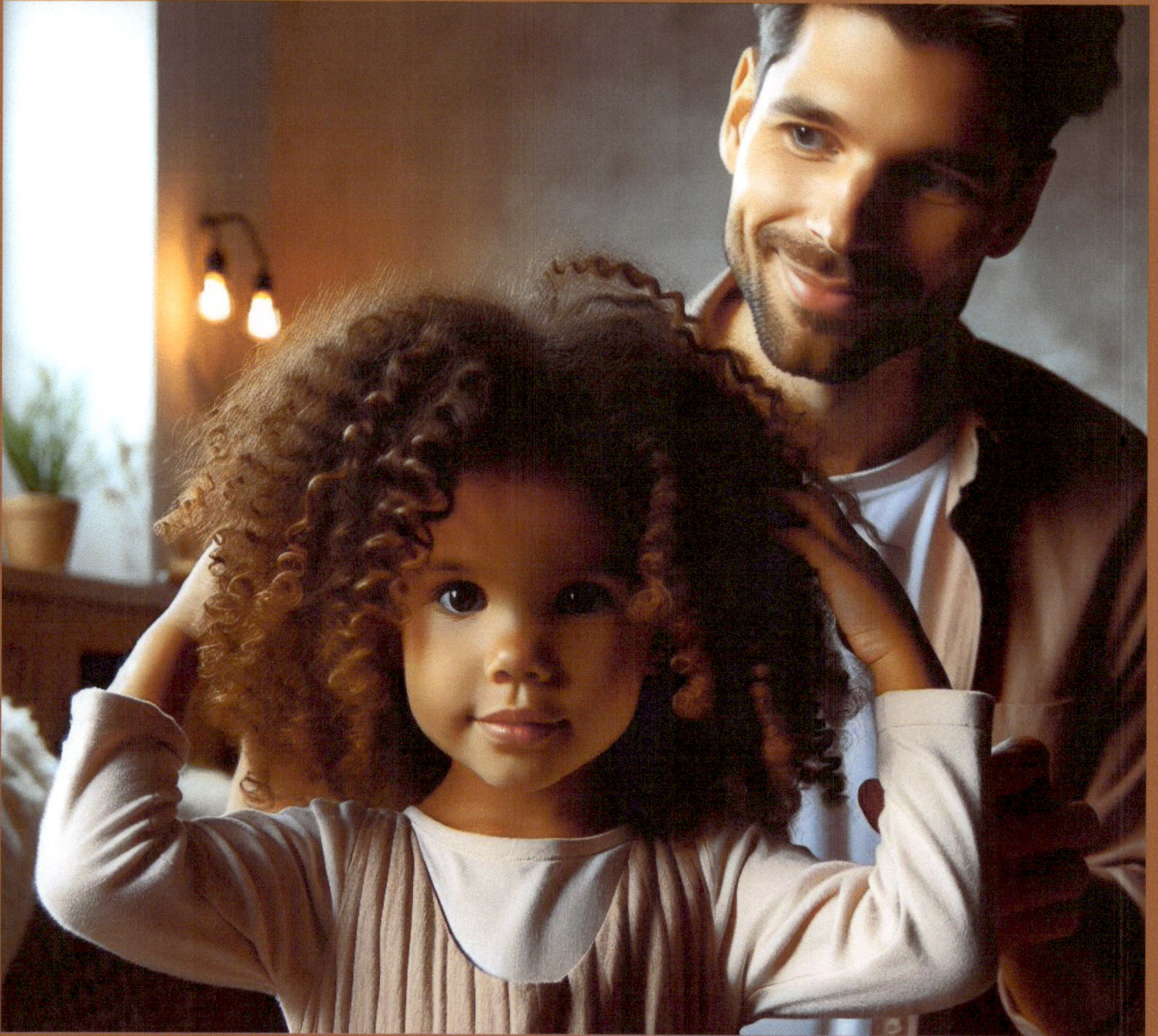

"Why is my hair curly when yours is straight?" I ask.

My dad smiles and says, "Because it's part of who you are. Your curls are beautiful, and I'm learning how to take care of them with you."

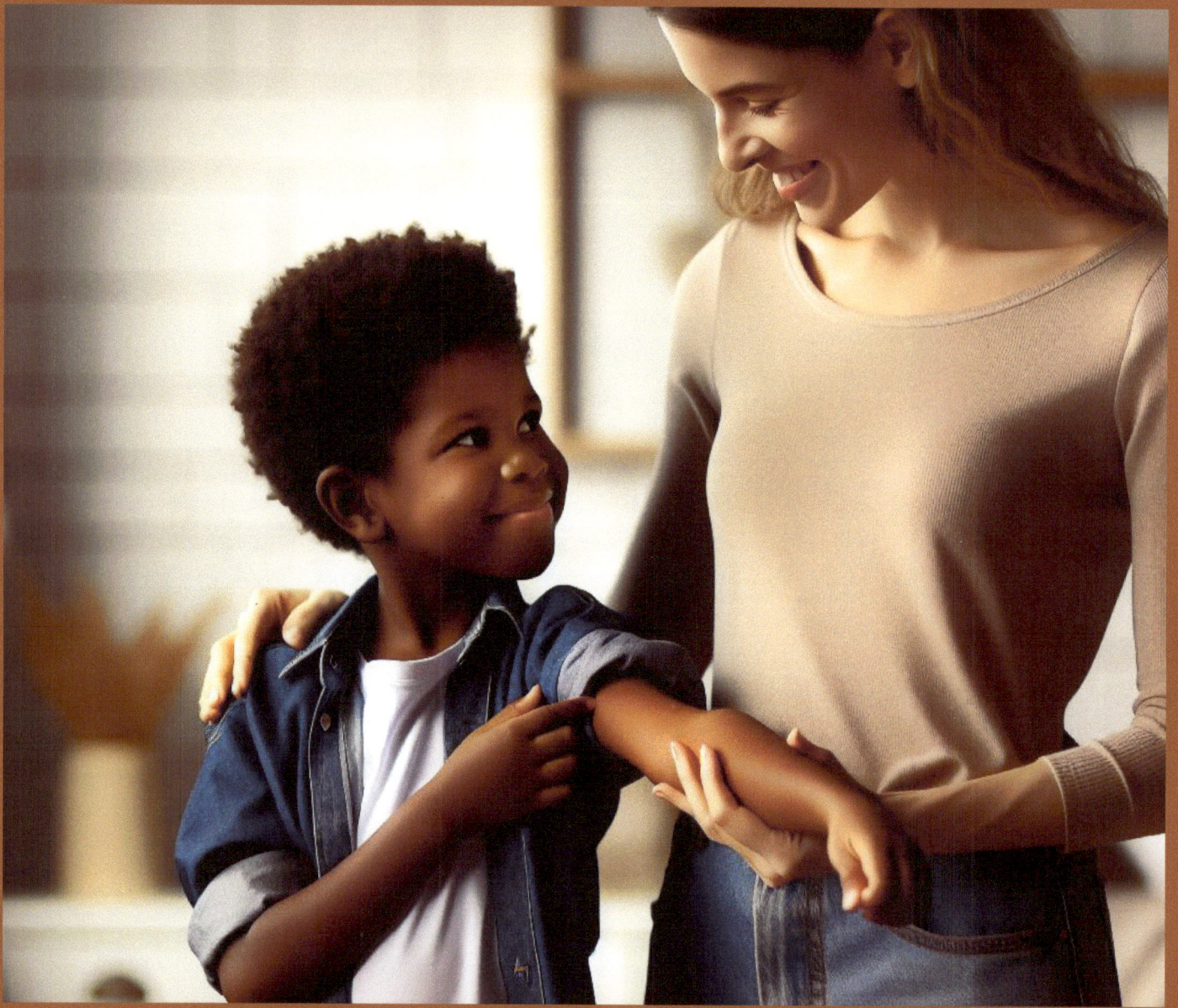

I also wonder about my skin.

It's darker than my parent's and doesn't turn pink in the sun like theirs does. People sometimes ask if I'm adopted, which makes me feel confused. Mom tells me my skin is beautiful!

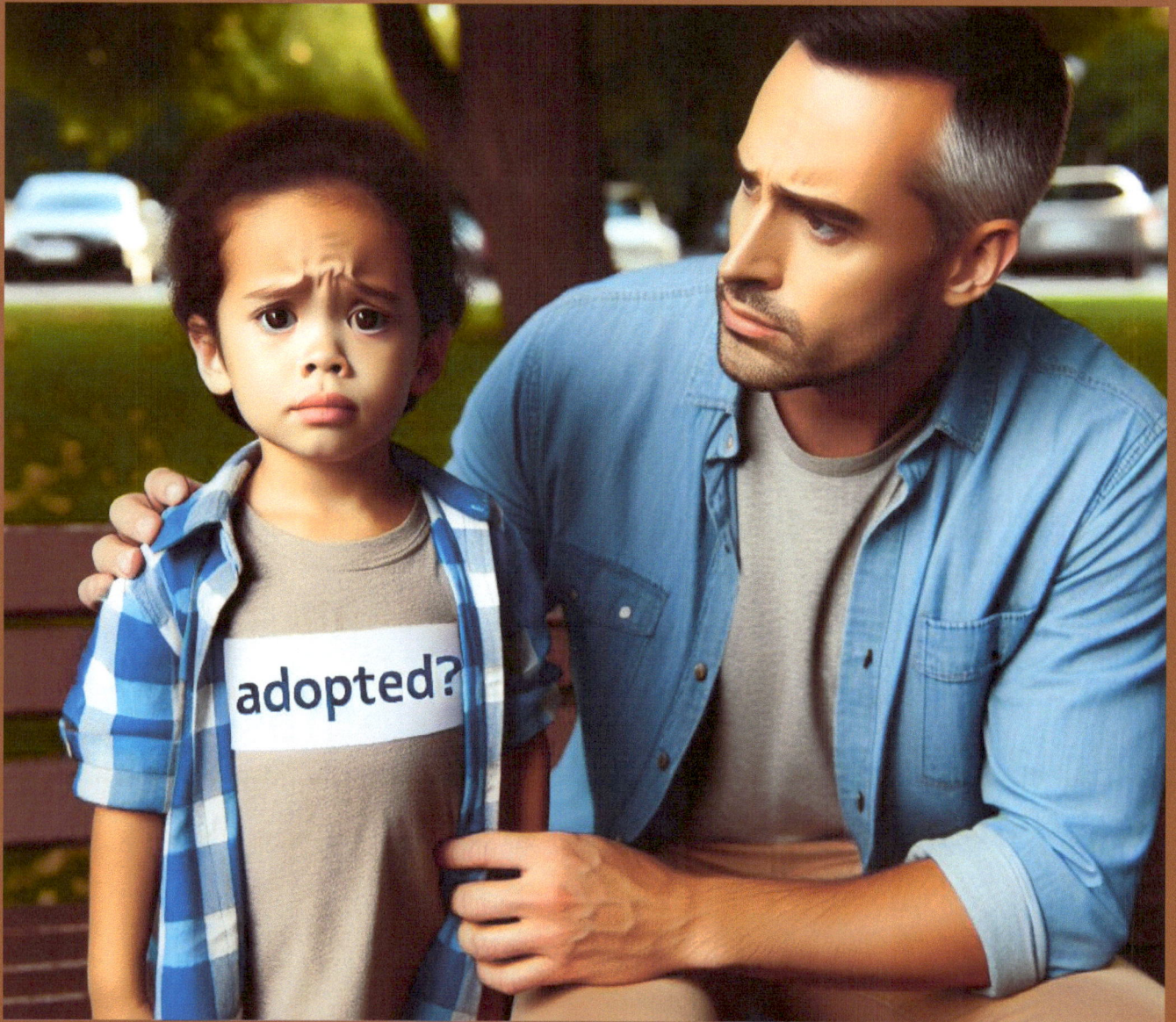

"Why do people ask me if I'm adopted?" I ask.

My dad sighs and says, "Sometimes people don't understand that families can look different. But you are mine, and I am yours. That's what matters most."

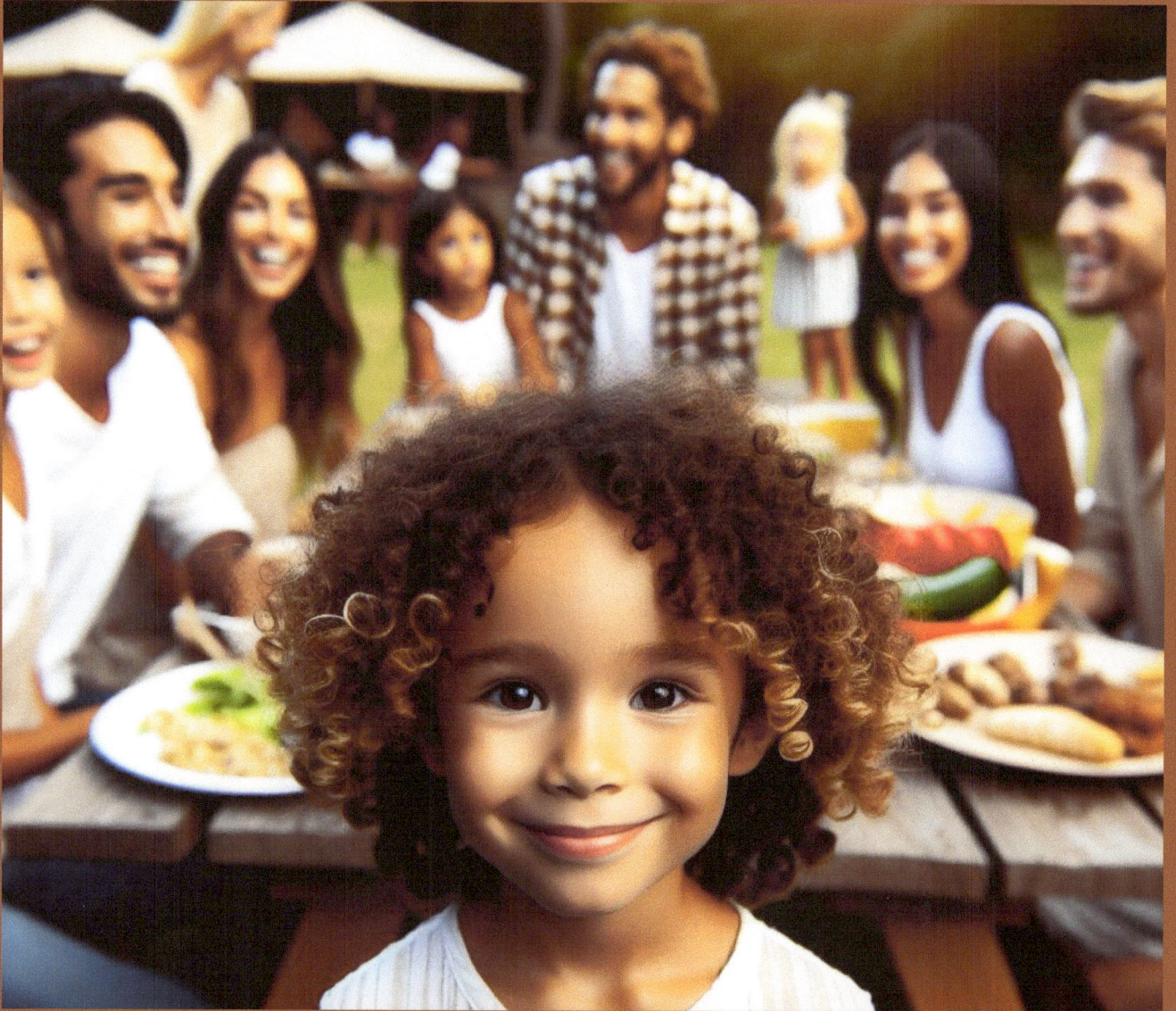

Sometimes, when I go to family gatherings,
I feel like I don't quite fit in.

My cousins all look alike, and their hair is easy to comb. No one ever asks them questions about where they belong.

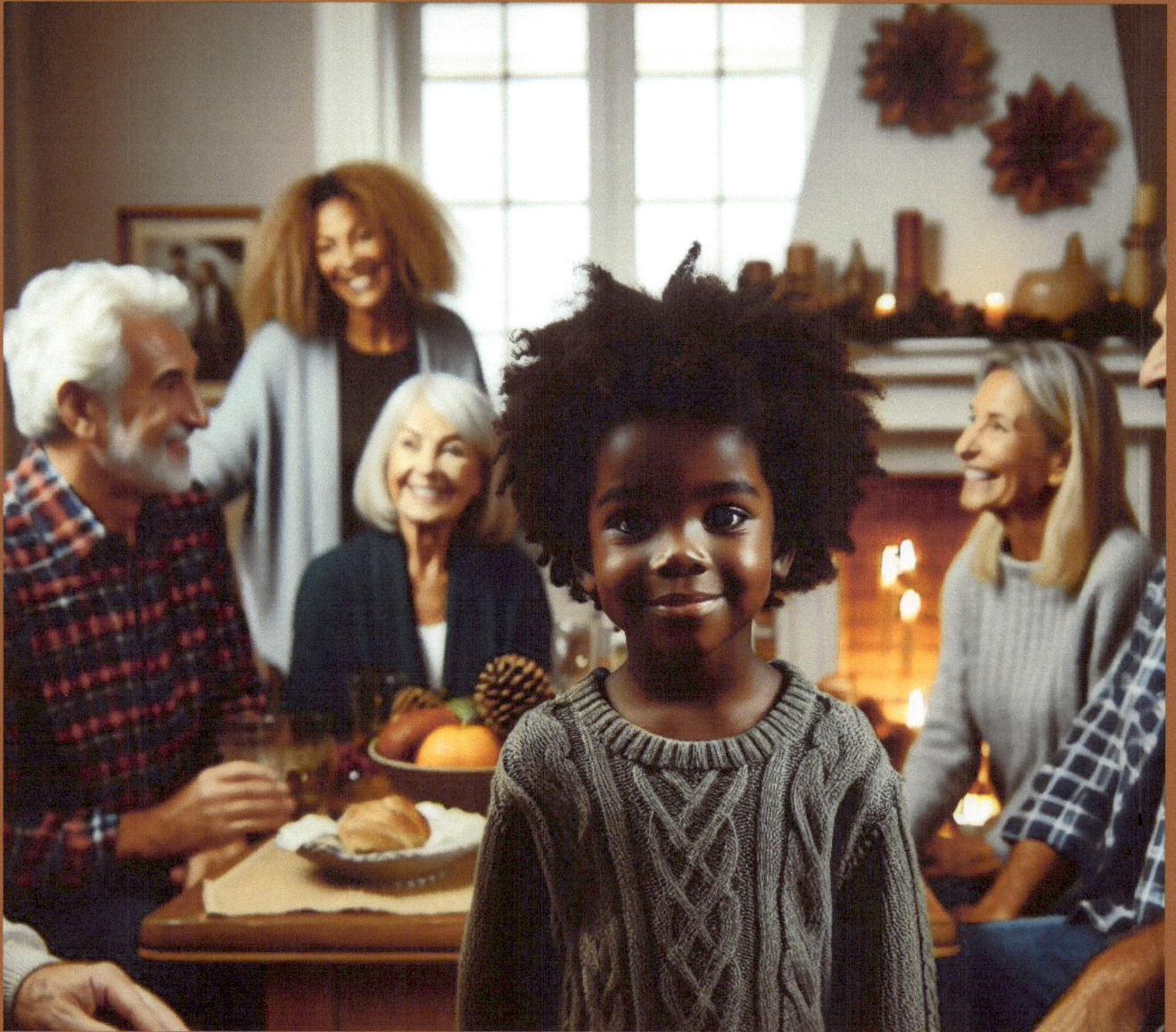

Sometimes, when I'm with my family, I feel like I stand out.

Most of them don't have my hair or my skin, and I wonder if they truly see all of me. Everyone is kind and loving, but it's still hard when I don't see anyone else who looks like me. I know they care, but sometimes I wish someone understood what it feels like to be the only one.

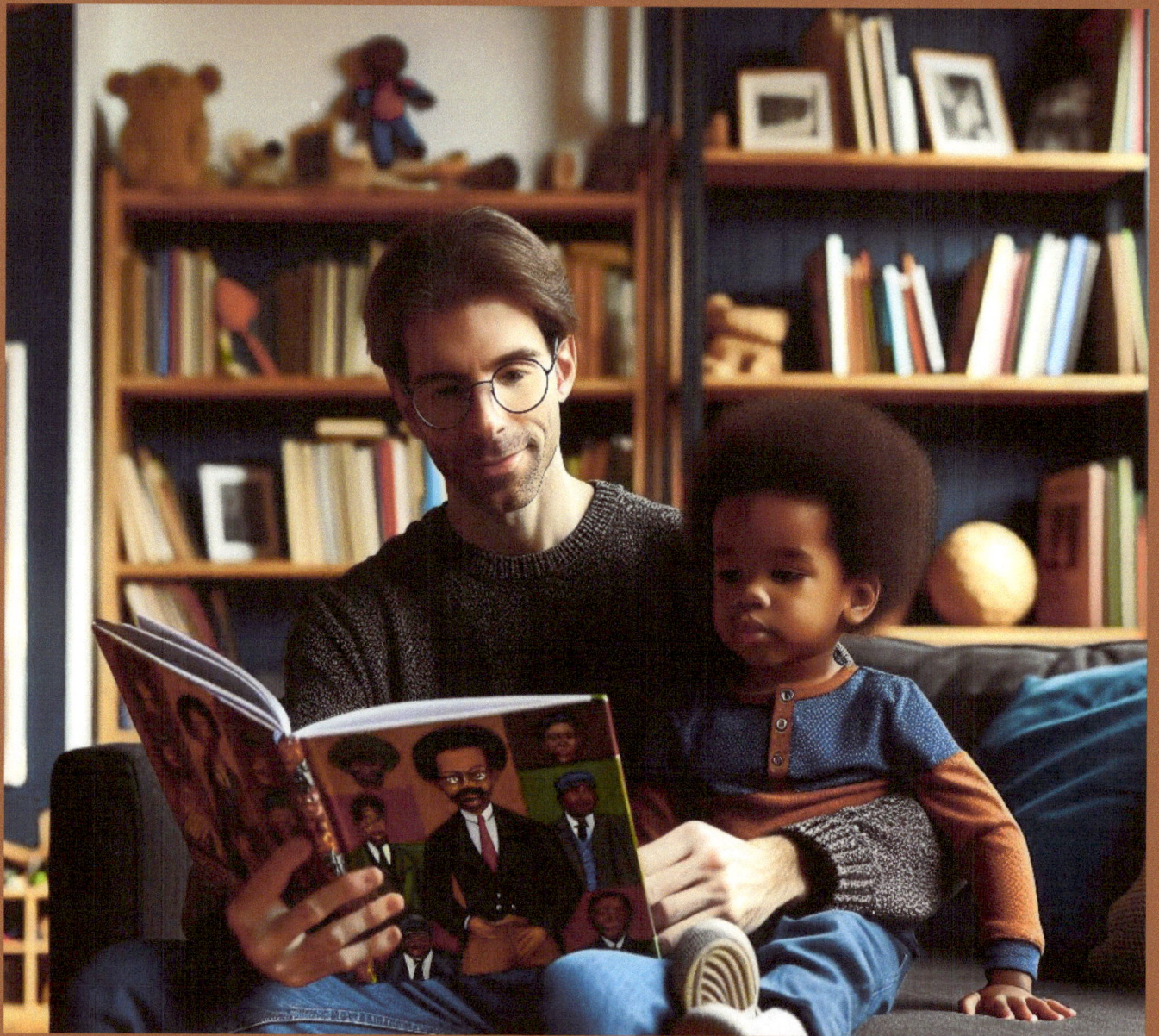

But my dad reminds me that being different isn't a
bad thing—it's something to celebrate!

"Your Blackness is something special," he says. "And I want to learn about it with you."

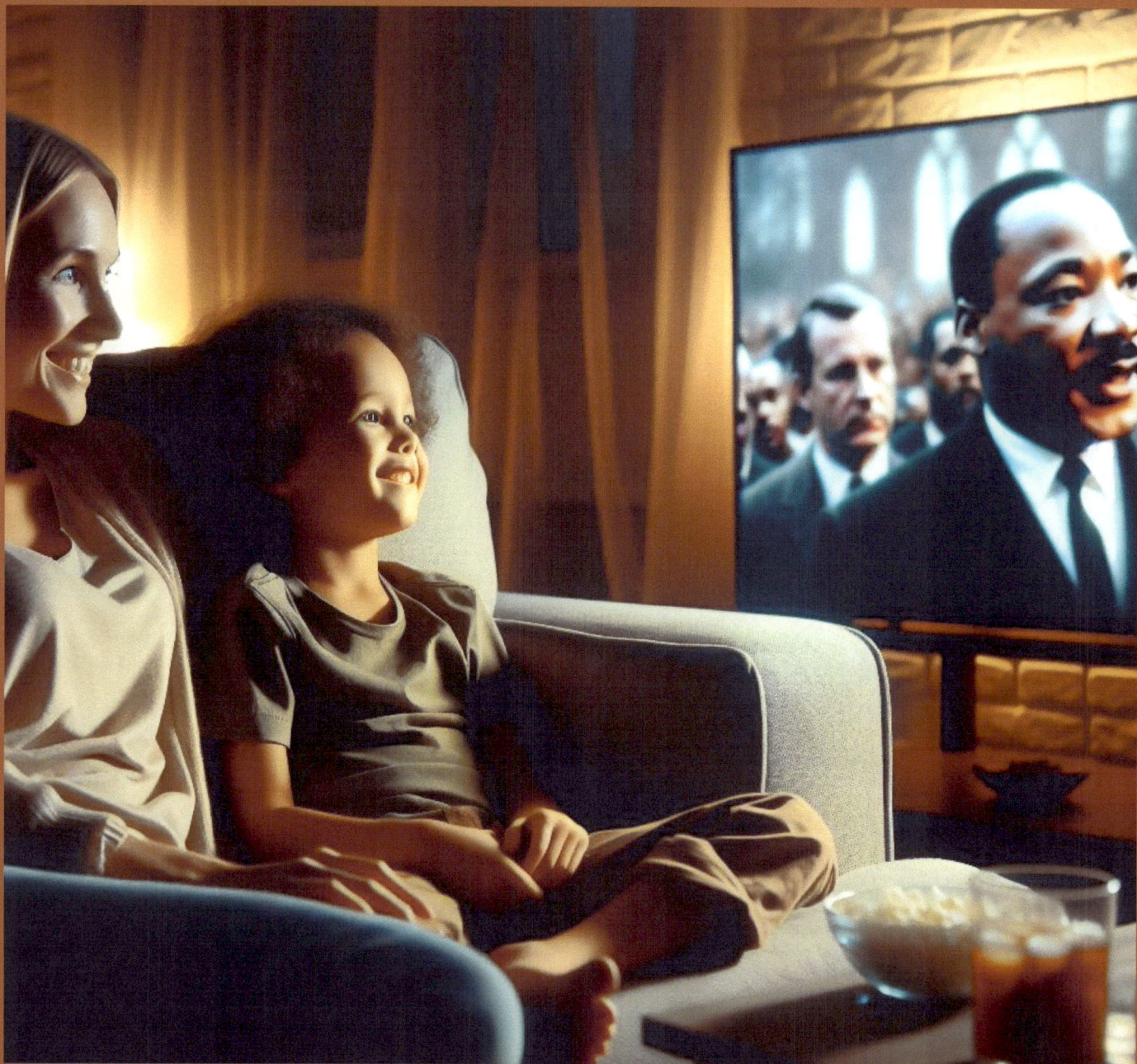

So, we start learning together.

We read books about amazing Black leaders, artists, and scientists. We watch movies where the heroes look like me. And we talk about what it means to be Black.

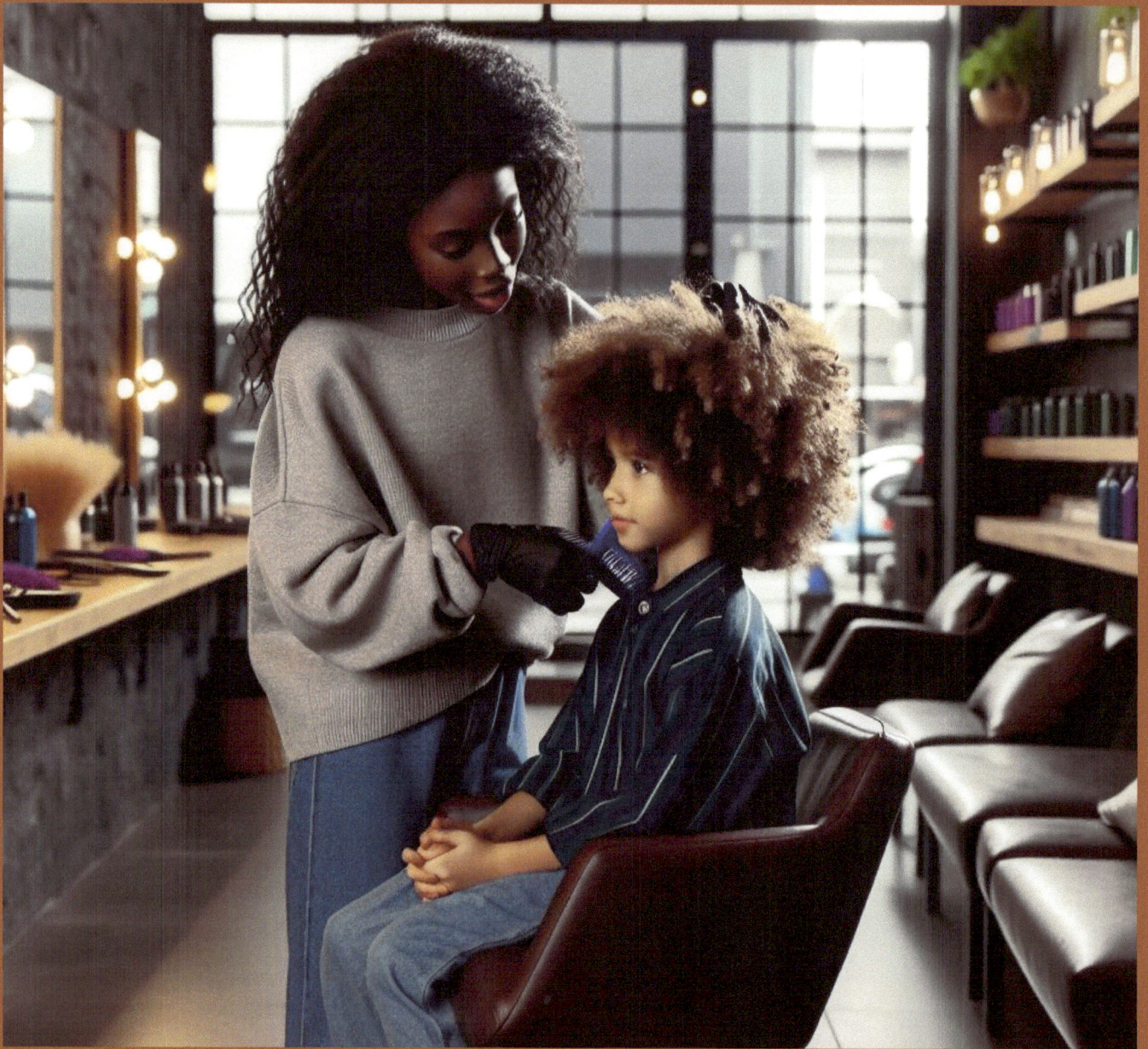

My mom also helps me meet other Black people who can teach me about my culture.

I meet barbers and hairstylists who know exactly what to do with my curls.
I make friends who share my experiences.

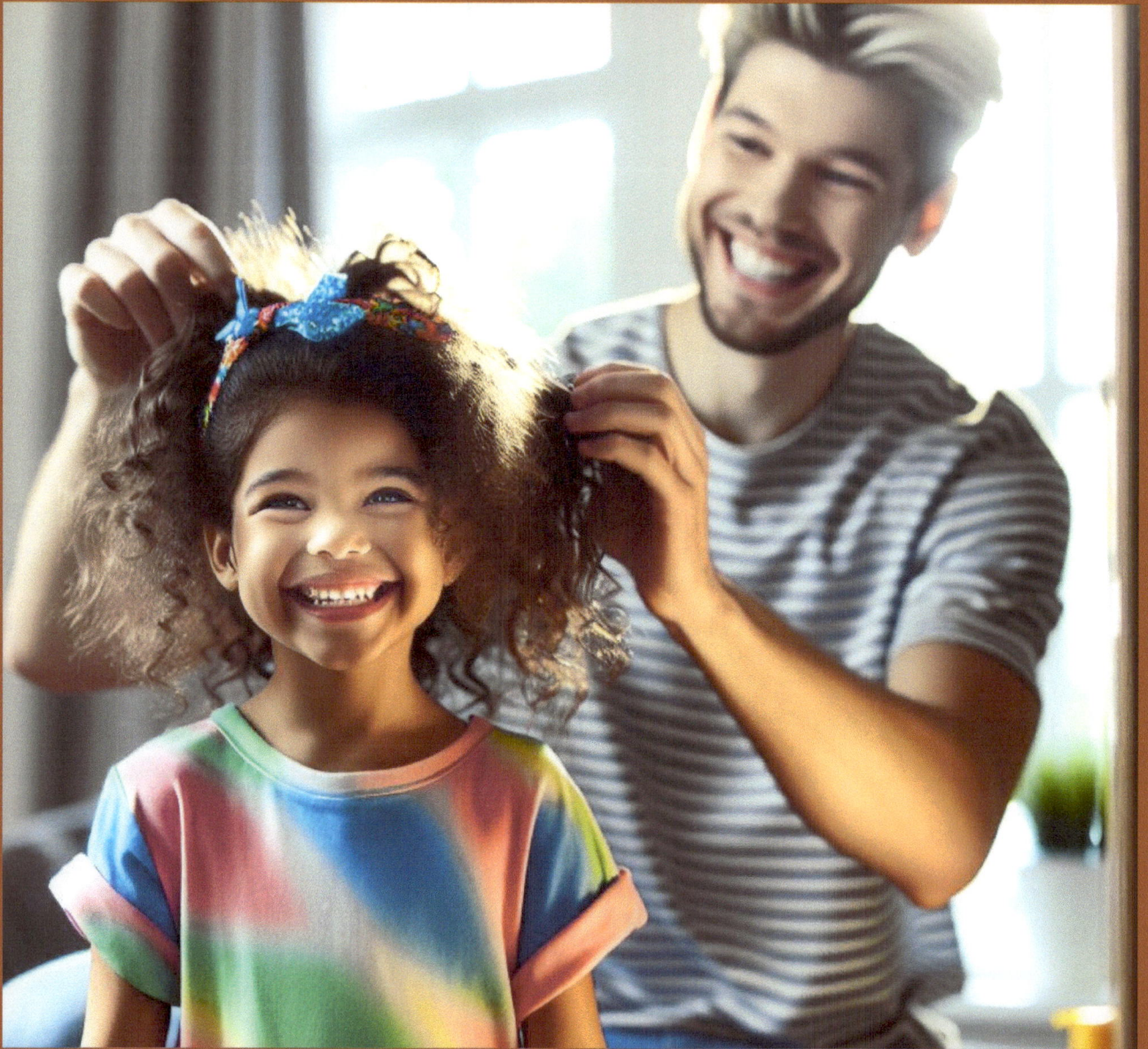

My hair is special.
My hair is my crown, and I wear it with pride!

It curls, coils, and stretches in ways that are all my own. My dad may not have hair like mine, but he learn with me. Together, we try different styles, find the right products, and make sure my hair stays healthy and strong.

**My hair is my crown,
and I wear it with pride!**

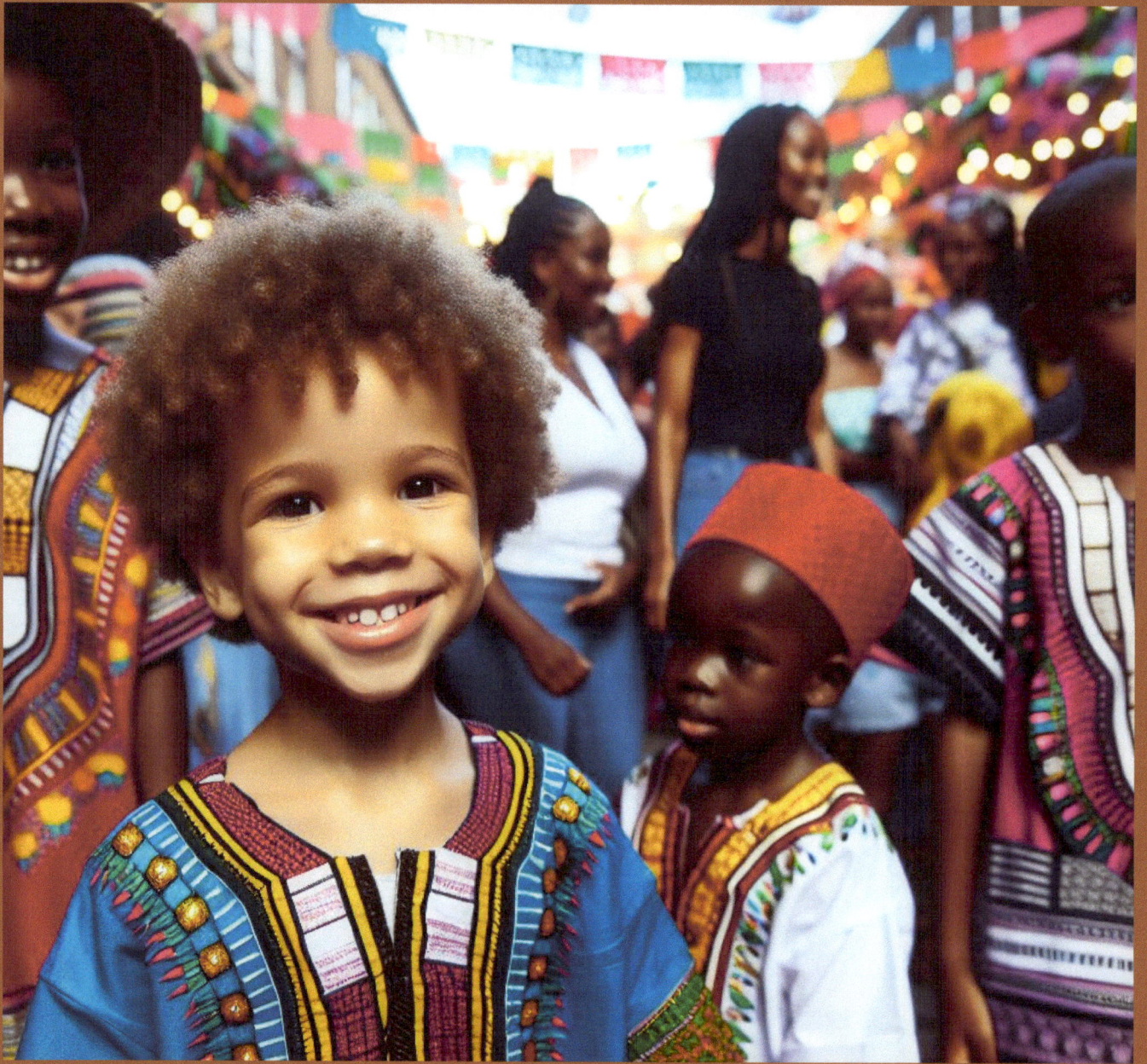

My mom and dad take me to places

where people look like me...

They take me to festivals, museums, and community events.
At first, I feel shy, but then I see other kids with hair like mine, and I feel at home.

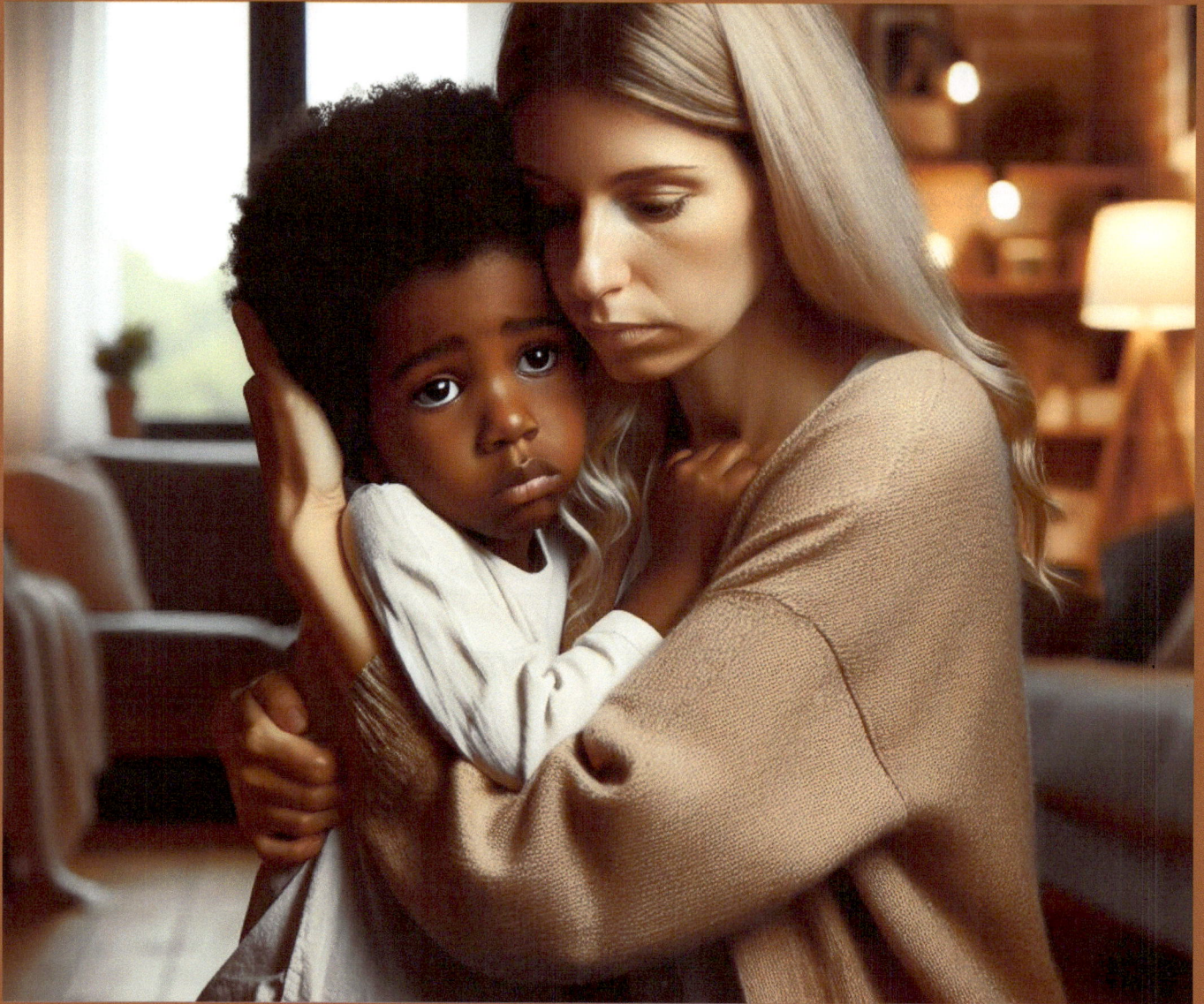

My mom listens to me when I feel left out...

...and stands up for me when people do not understand.

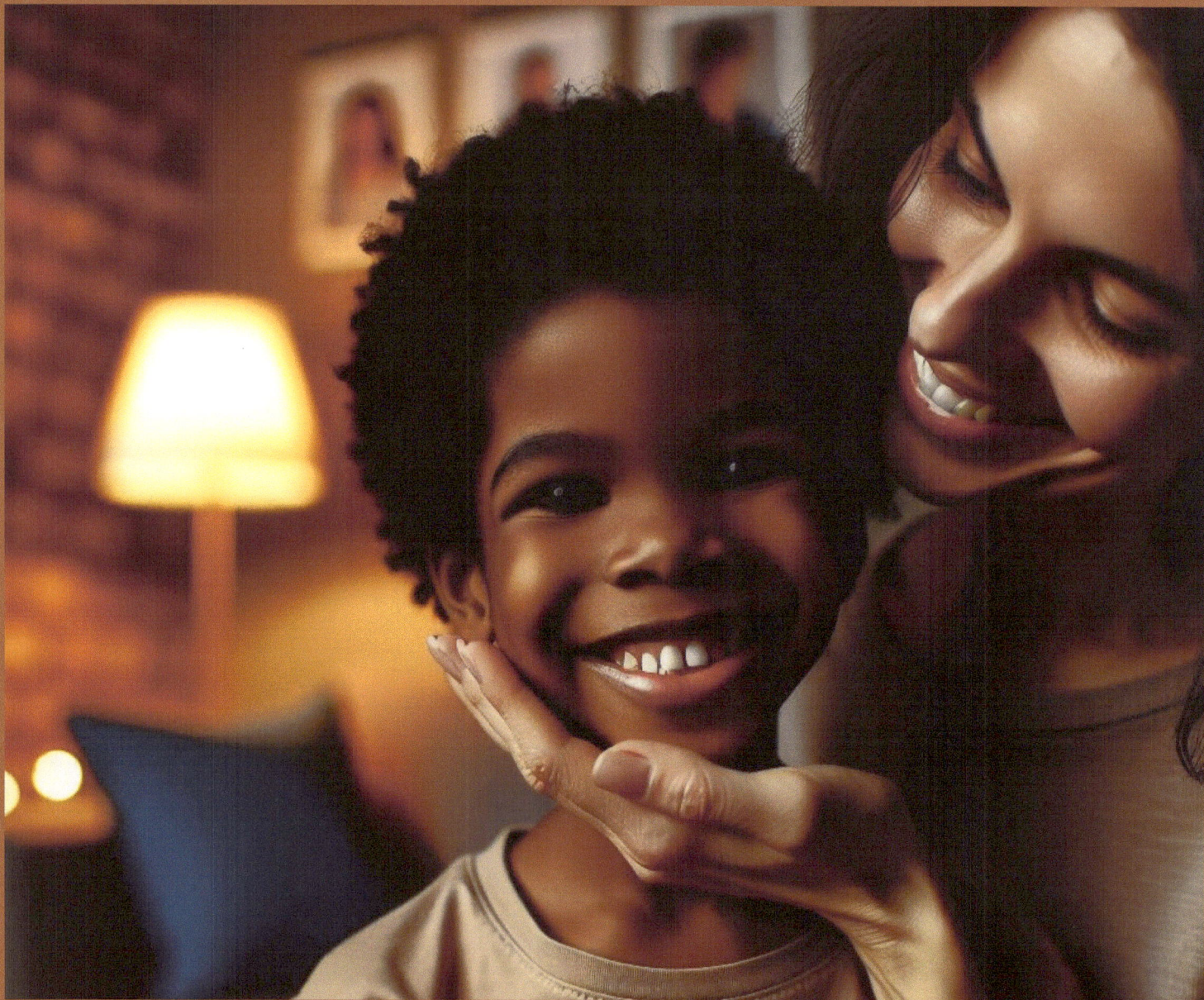

Sometimes, people ask me questions about my family.
They may wonder why my mom or dad looks different from me.

But to me, love is what makes a family, not how we look. My parent(s) may not share my skin or my curls, but they share their heart, their care, and their love. And that's what matters most.

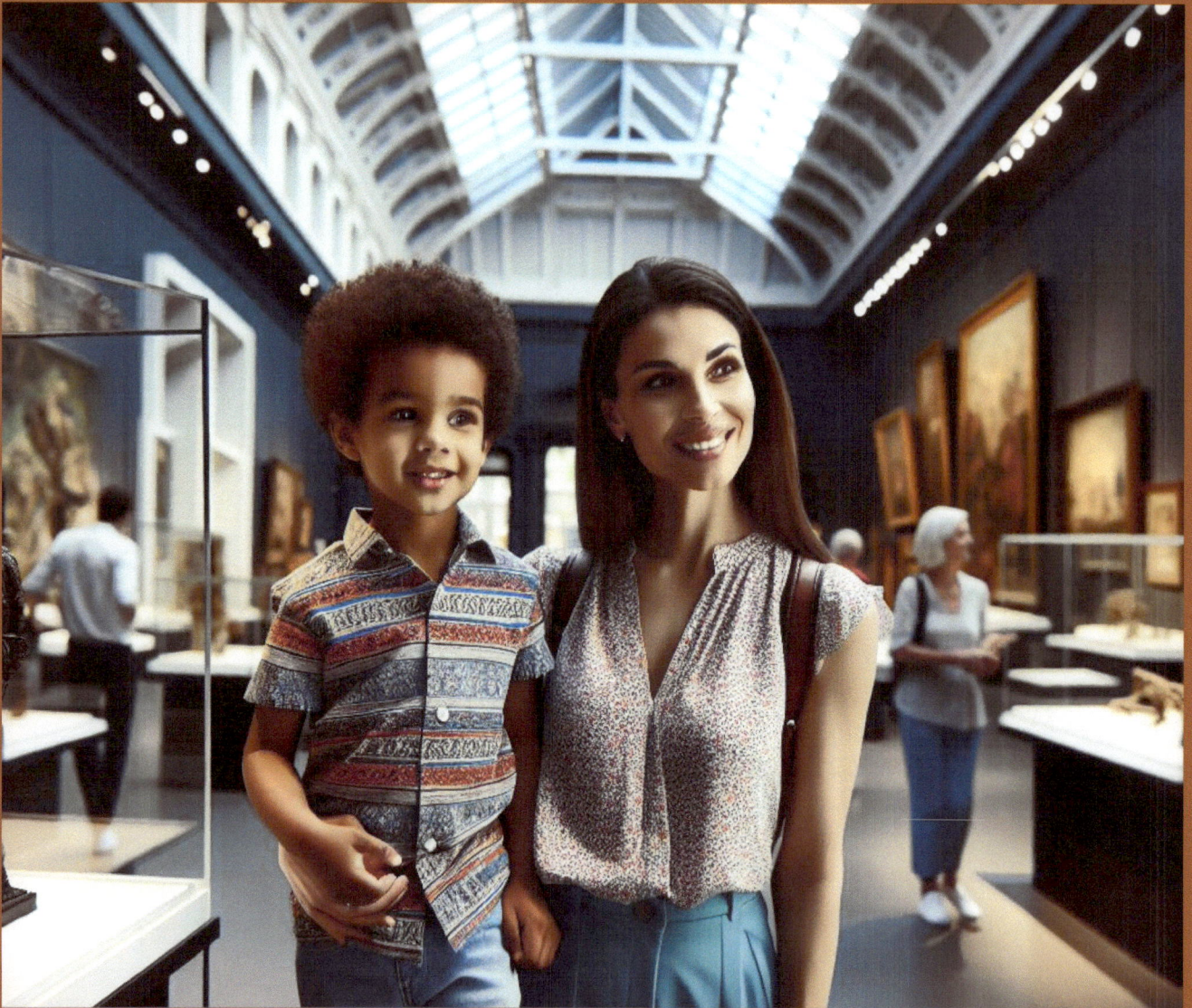

Today, my parent took me to a museum
to learn more about my history.

Walking through the halls, I saw paintings, sculptures, and artifacts that told stories of people who looked like me. Some were inventors, artists, and leaders. I felt proud knowing that my ancestors were strong, creative, and brave. Even though my parent doesn't share my history, they want me to know where I come from, and that means a lot to me.

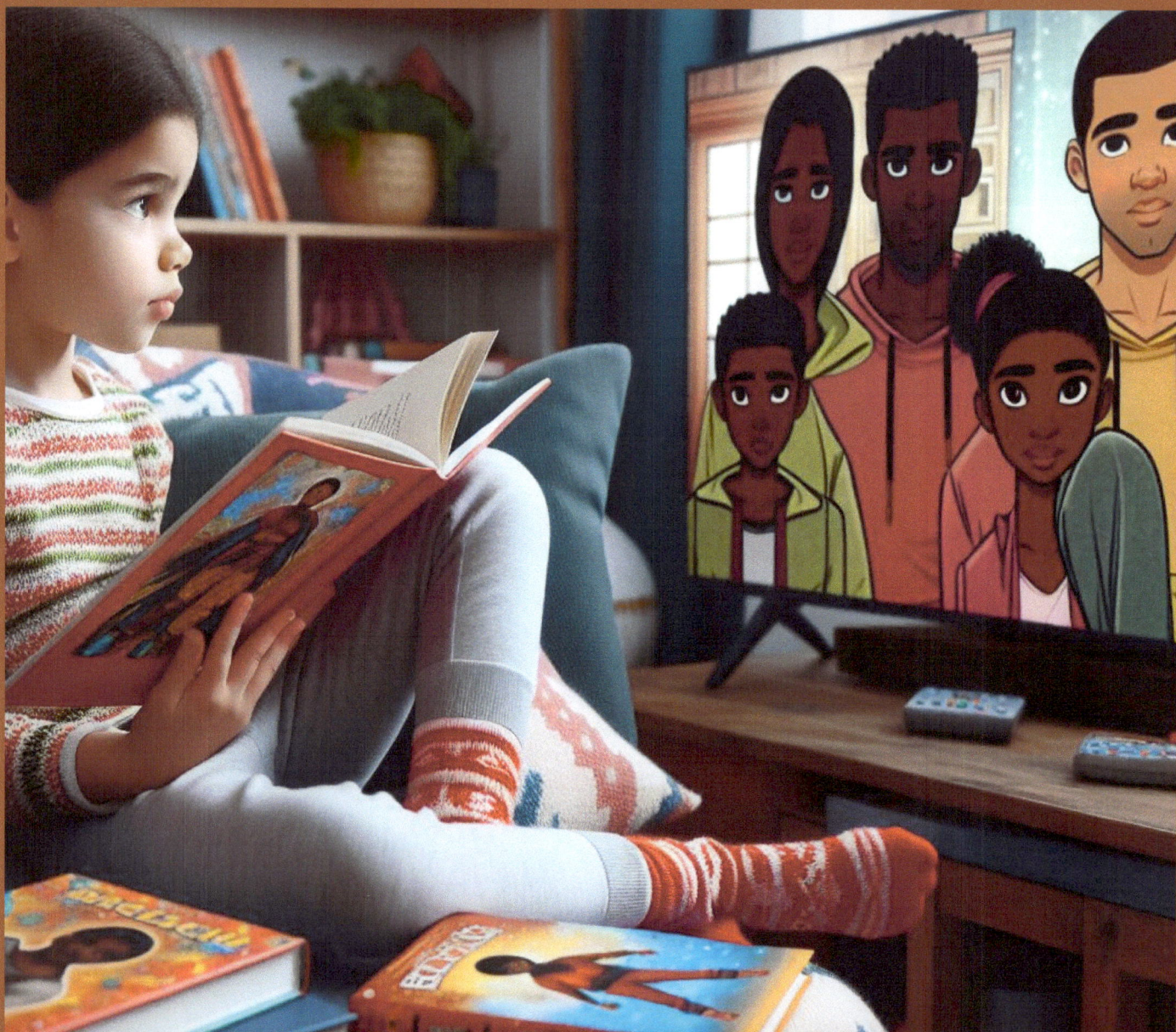

At home, we read books and watch shows where the characters look like me.

I see Black heroes, magical girls with curls like mine, and families who remind me of my own. These stories make me feel seen and proud. My parent helps me find books and shows that celebrate Black voices, history, and joy. It feels good to know that I belong in every story, too.

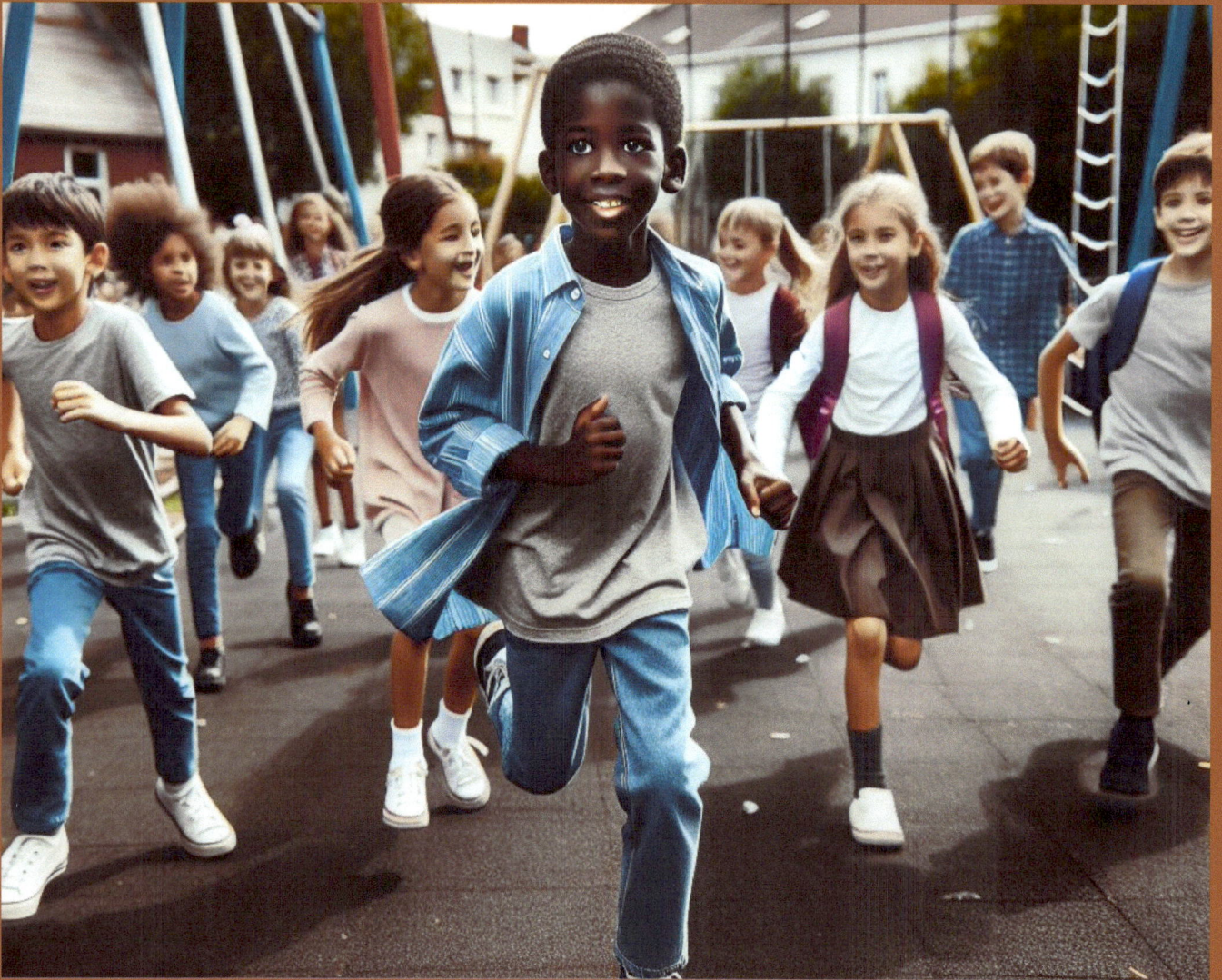

I sometimes wondered if I really fit in.

But now, I know that I belong—on the playground, in the classroom, and anywhere I go. I don't have to change who I am to be accepted. I can be proud of my skin, my voice, and my story. I run, laugh, and play just like everyone else. I am part of the world around me.

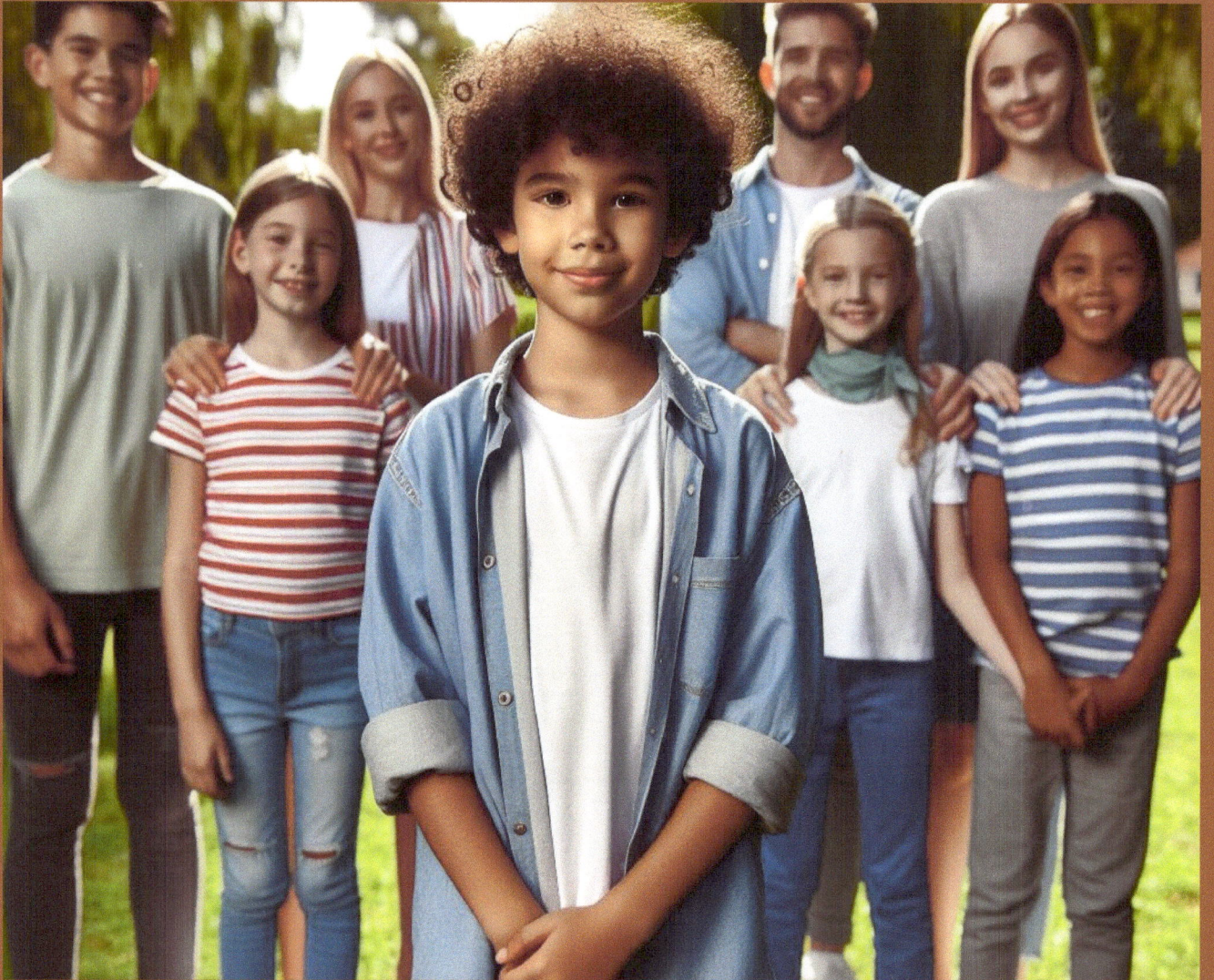

Even when people don't understand me,
I know who I am.

I am learning to stand tall, speak up, and feel proud. Being Black is a part of me— just like my kindness, my talents, and my dreams. I don't need to explain everything about myself to be accepted. I carry my truth with confidence wherever I go.

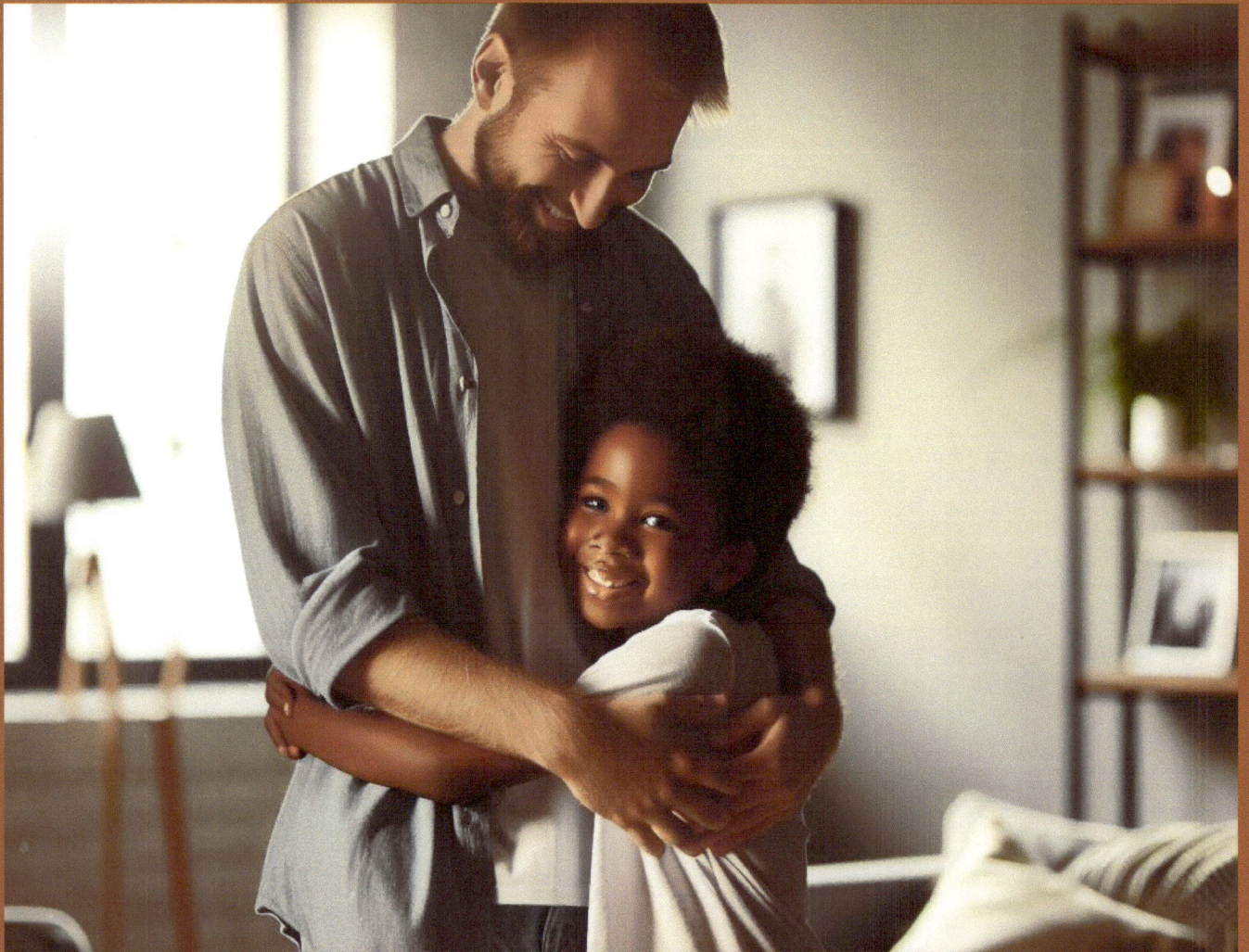

Being Black in my family might look different from what some people expect—but love lives here.

We don't have to look the same to care for each other deeply.

My parent supports me, learns with me, and makes sure I feel safe and celebrated. In our home, love wraps around me like a warm hug.

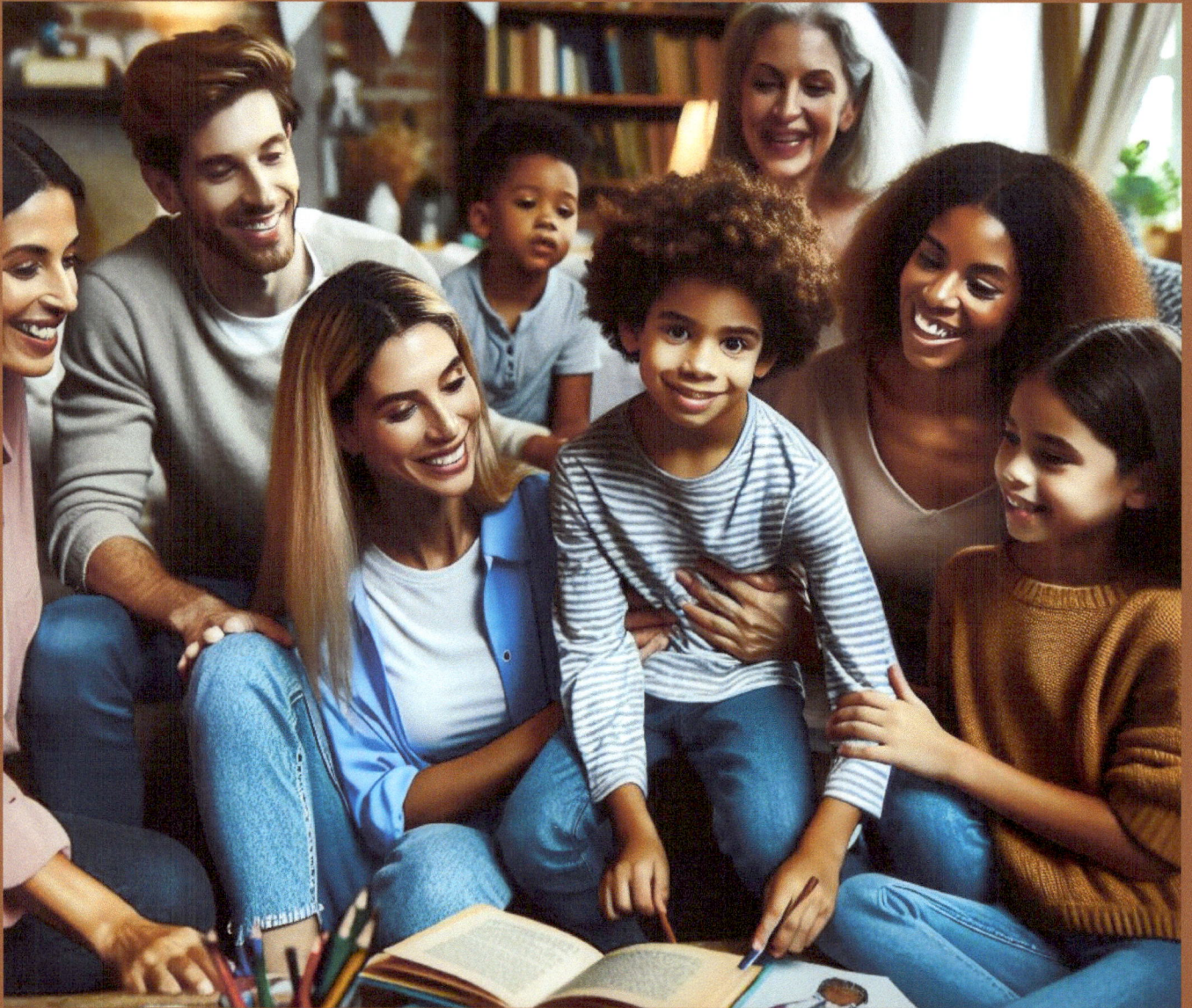

In my family, we learn from each other.

We read, ask questions, and talk about things that matter—like identity, culture, and kindness. My parent doesn't know everything about being Black, but they try to learn with me. They ask for help, listen with their heart, and grow alongside me. That's what makes our bond even stronger.

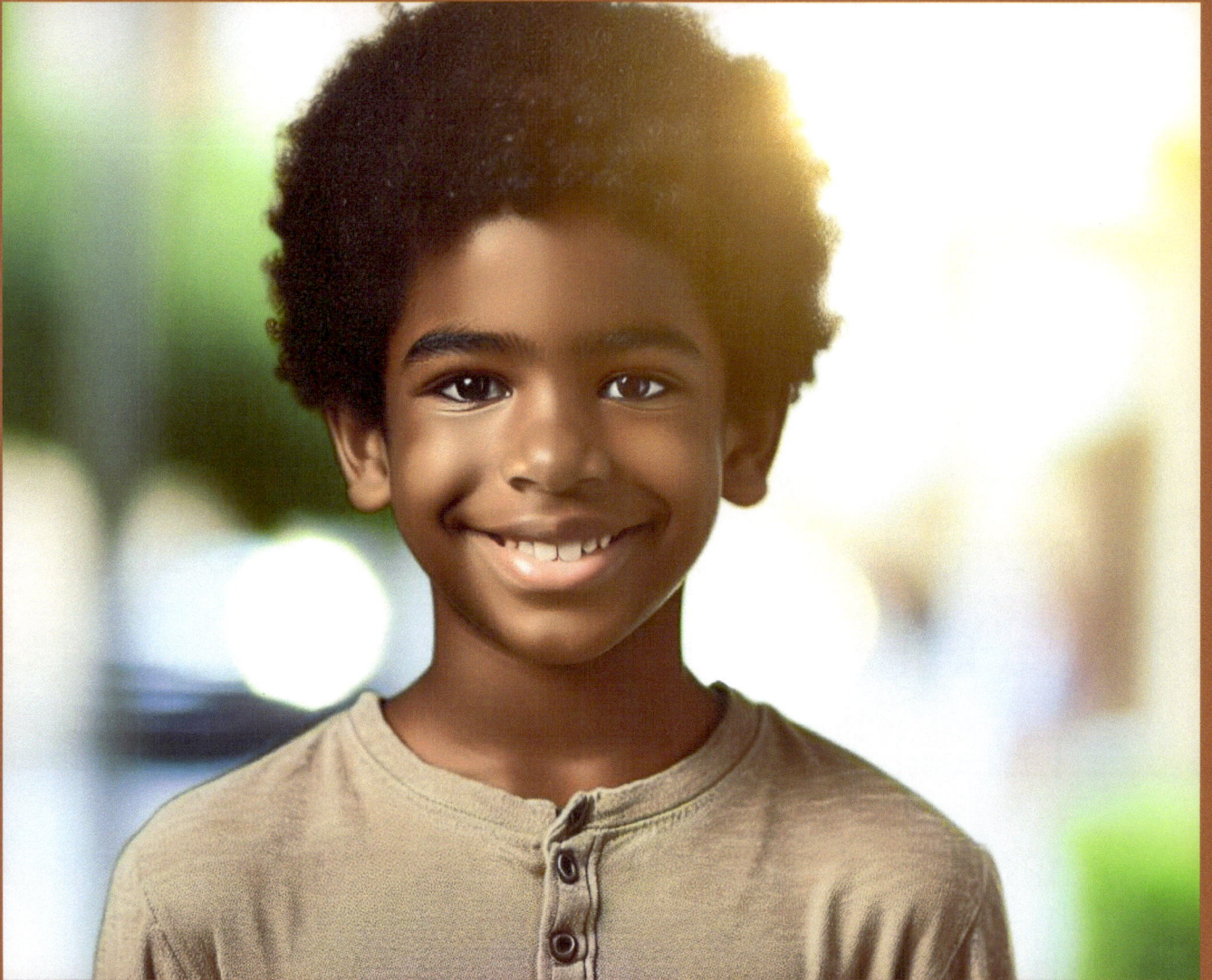

I am proud of who I am. I don't need to hide, change, or shrink to make others feel comfortable.

My skin, my hair, my voice, and my story are all important.

I can speak with confidence, walk with pride, and shine just by being myself.

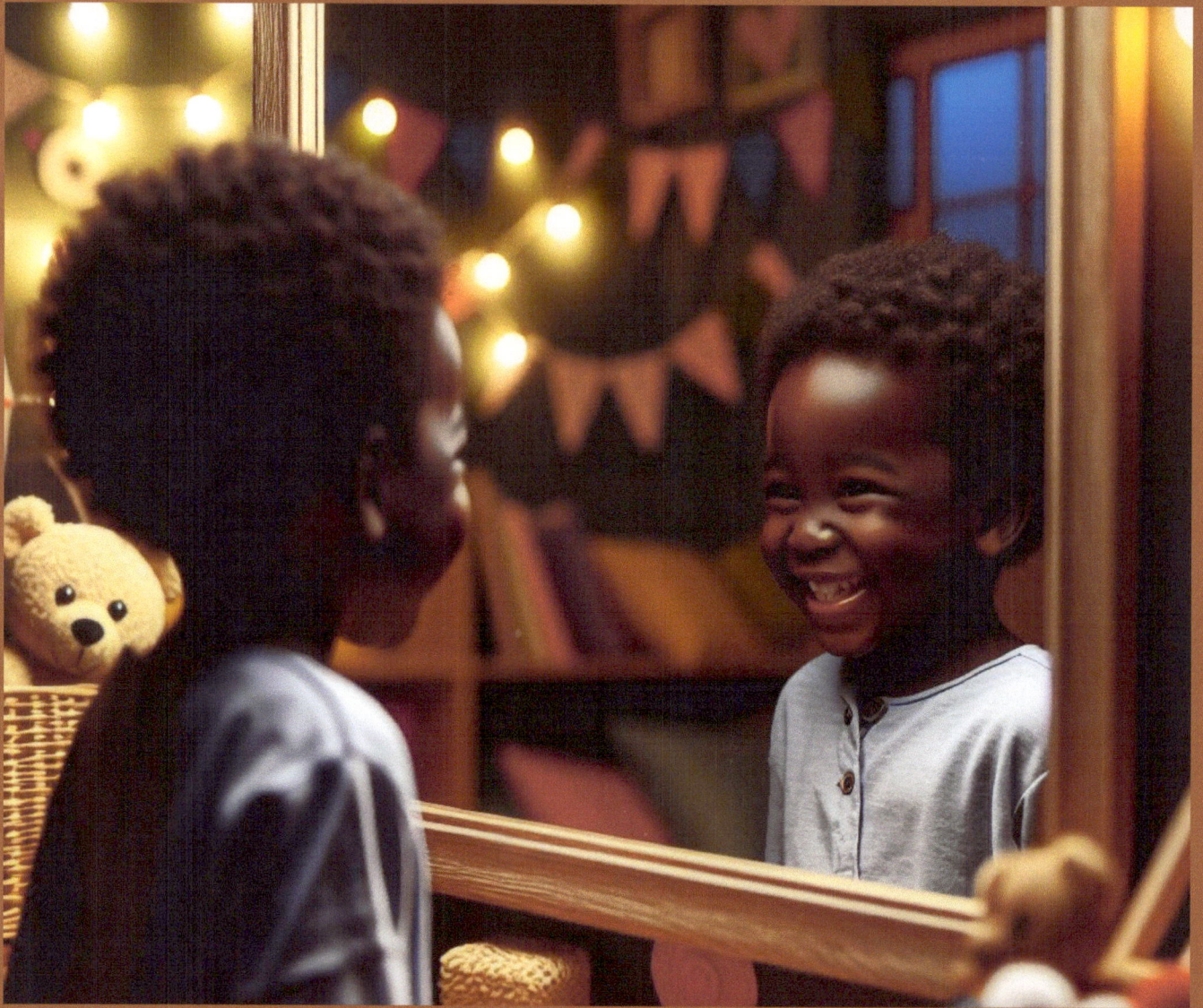

When I look in the mirror, I see someone smart, kind, and full of life.

I see skin kissed by sunshine, hair that rises like a crown, and eyes that hold dreams. I remind myself: I am Black. I am loved. I am enough—just the way I am.

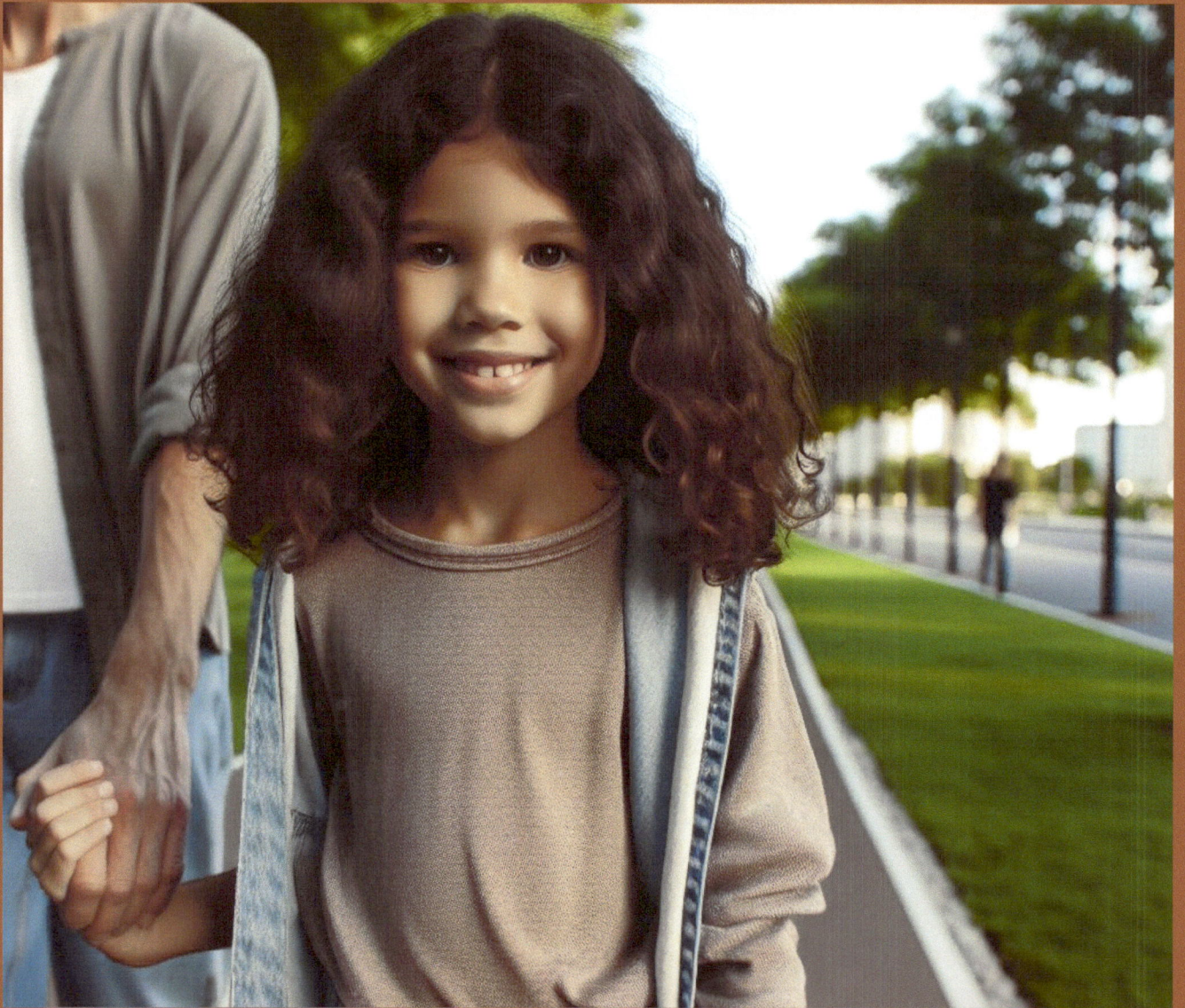

When I walk through the world, I carry love with me.

The love from my parent, who holds my hand and walks beside me. The love from my culture, my ancestors, and my story. I am not alone, even when I feel different. I am surrounded by love, and that love gives me strength.

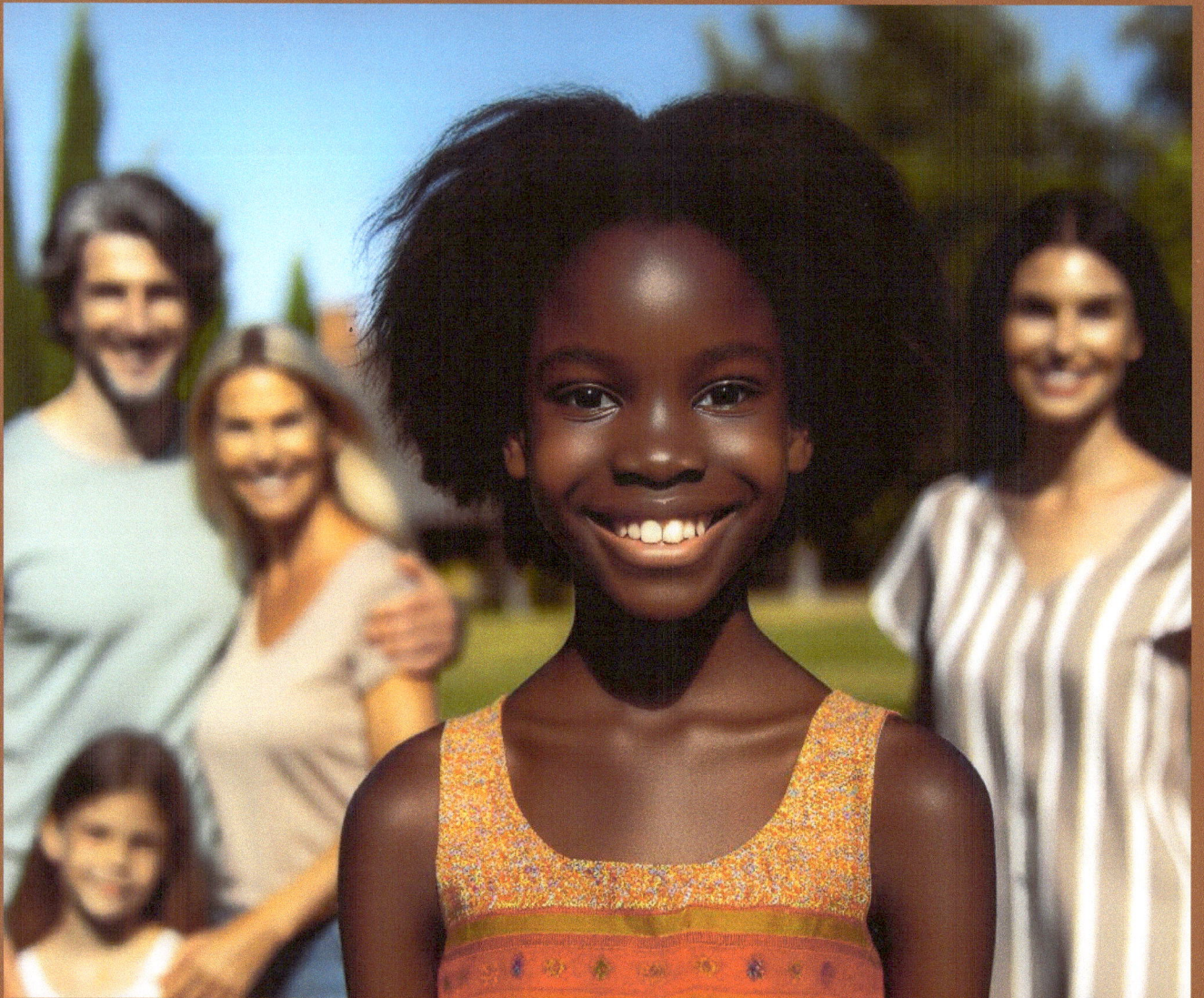

Being Black in my family is a journey.

Sometimes it's joyful, sometimes it's hard. But every step teaches me something about who I am. My family may not look like me, but they love me, learn with me, and stand by me. I am Black. I am brilliant. I am bold. And no matter where I go or who I'm with—**I belong**.

I am seen. I am supported. I am strong. I am exactly who I'm meant to be.

Dear Parent or Caregiver,

Thank you for walking alongside your child through Being Black in My Family. This book was created to reflect the experiences of mixed-race children raised in non-Black households—children who are learning to understand their Black identity in the context of love, difference, and growth.

The pages you've just read were designed to help your child feel seen, celebrated, and affirmed. The next section offers an opportunity for deeper reflection. You'll find questions meant to guide thoughtful conversations between you and your child—conversations that may be joyful, curious, emotional, or challenging.

We encourage you to explore these reflection questions together. Give your child space to express what they're thinking and feeling. If they're unsure, let them know it's okay. This isn't about having perfect answers—it's about connection.
Be open. Be patient. Be present. These small moments can become powerful memories.

You don't need to have all the answers. What matters most is your willingness to listen, to learn, and to show your child that their identity is beautiful and important.

Thank you for choosing to grow with your child.

Thank you for choosing love.

"I am not half of anything.
I am whole."
— Unknown

"Your Blackness is beautiful, no matter
how others see it.
It's yours."
— Sol ☀

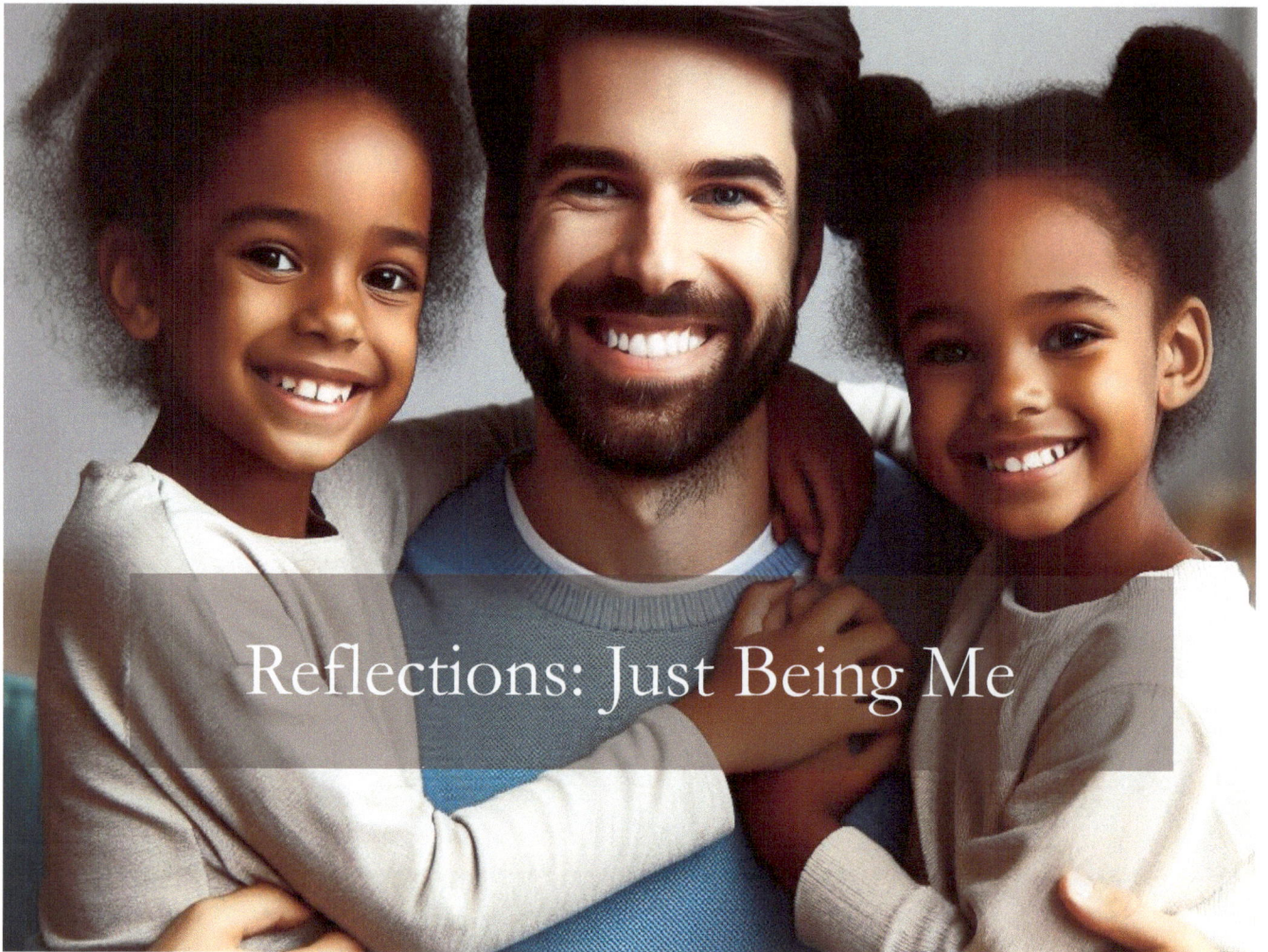

Reflections: Just Being Me

1. What does being Black mean to you right now?
2. What's one thing you love about your Blackness?
3. What's something new you've learned about your family or culture?
4. How do you feel when people don't understand your identity? What helps you feel strong in those moments?
5. Who is someone you can talk to when you have big questions or big feelings?

Reflections: Just Being Me

1. What does being Black mean to you right now?

2. What's one thing you love about your Blackness?

3. What's something new you've learned about your family or culture?

4. How do you feel when people don't understand your identity? What helps you feel strong in those moments?

5. Who is someone you can talk to when you have big questions or big feelings?

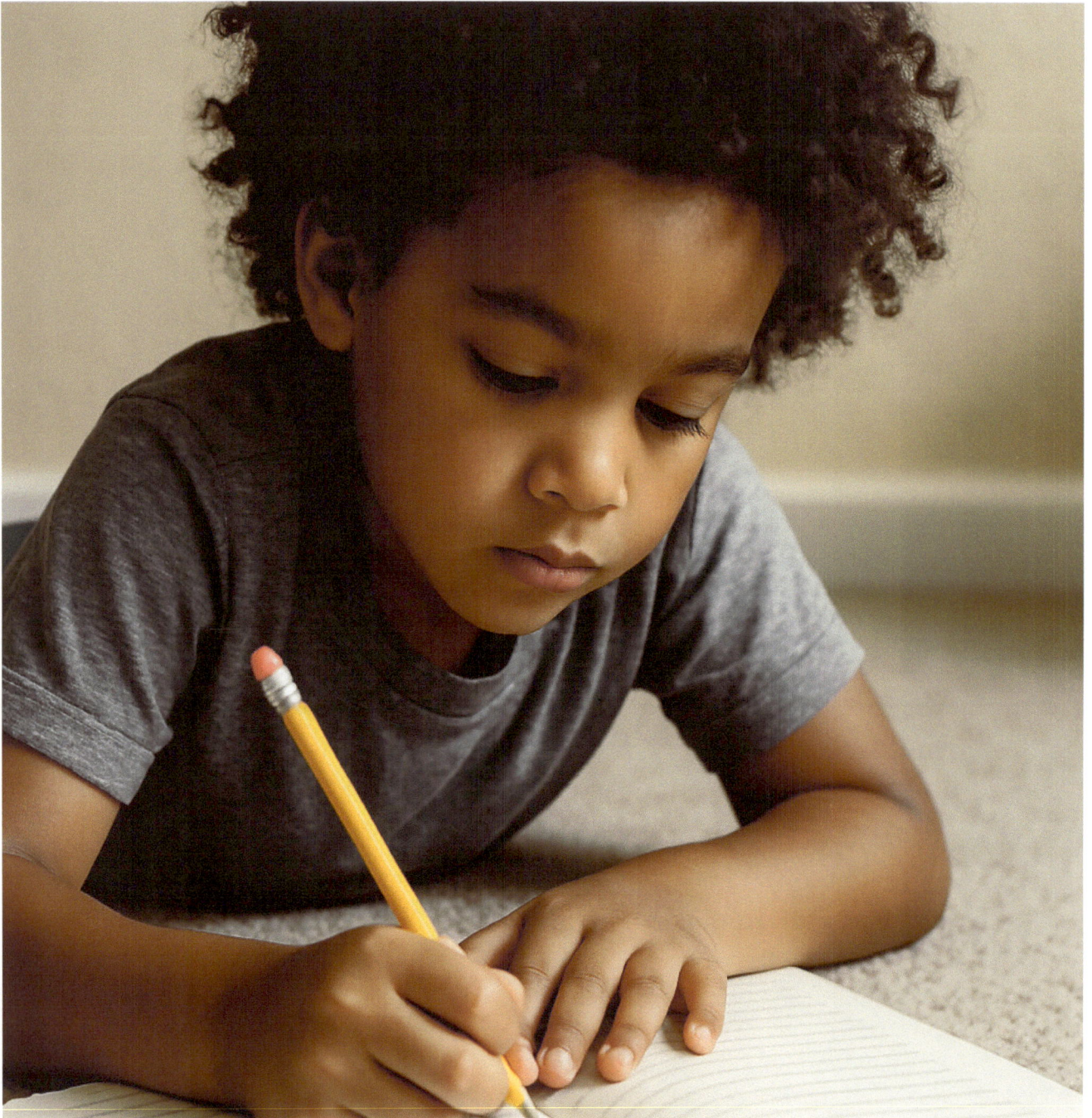

"Letter to Myself"

Write a short letter to your future self.
Tell them something you want them to remember about your identity,
your family, and how special you are.

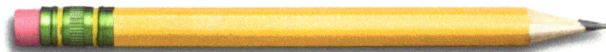

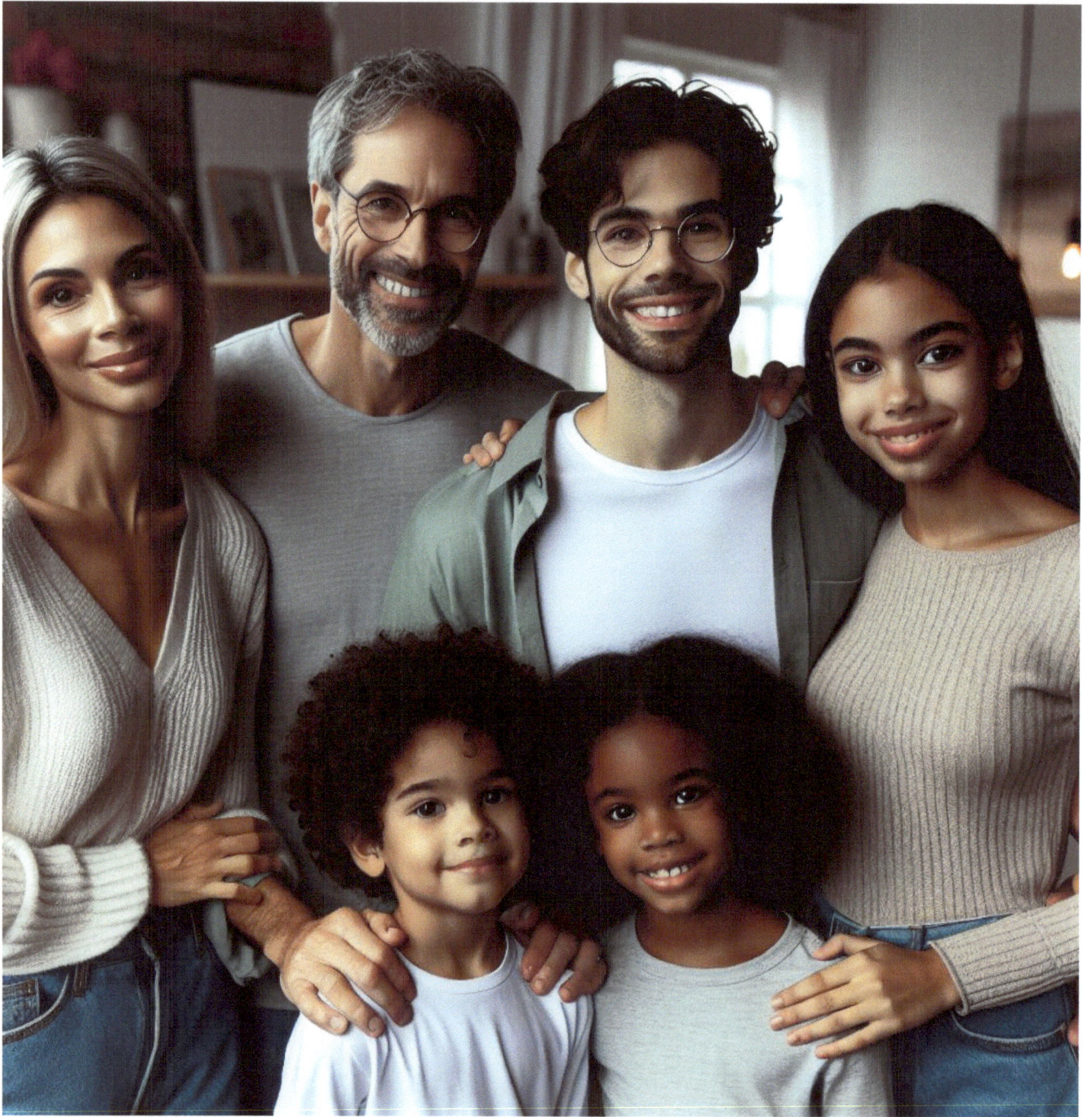

Page 62

"My Family, My Story" Collage

Draw or glue pictures of the people who matter to you.
You can include family, friends, ancestors, pets, or anyone else who makes you
feel loved and seen.

What does it mean to be Black in a family where not everyone looks like you?

In Being Black in My Family, young readers explore identity, belonging, and the beauty of their Blackness—even in spaces where it might feel invisible. Through honest reflections, heartfelt questions, and gentle storytelling, this book invites children to feel seen, supported, and proud of who they are.

Whether it's curly hair, deep questions, or learning about culture, this book helps children navigate the joy and complexity of growing up in a multiracial family—with love leading the way.

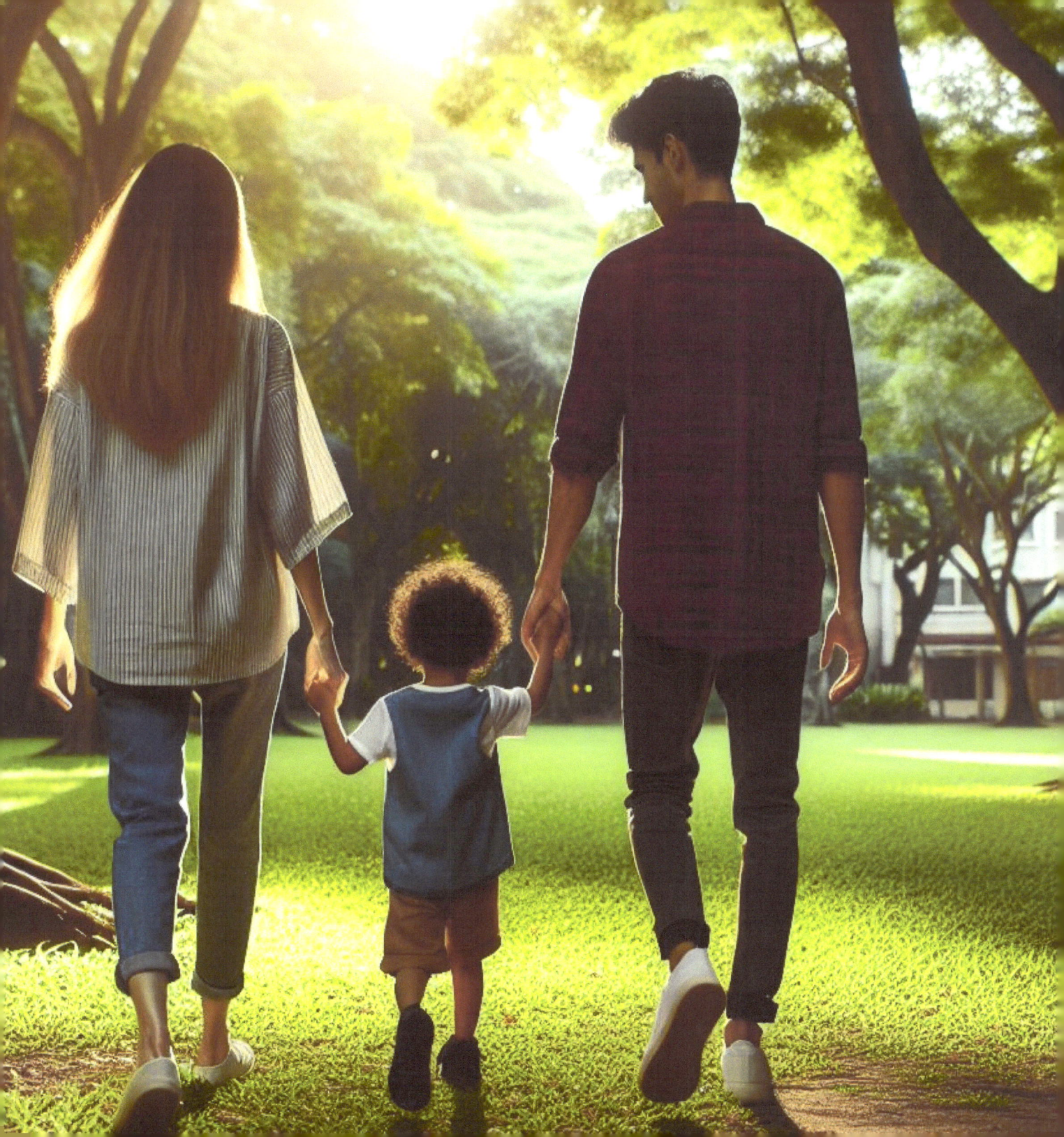

www.ingramcontent.com/pod-product-compliance
Lightning Source LLC
Chambersburg PA
CBHW060806270326
41927CB00002B/66